VOIGHT

VOIGHT

precision training
for body & mind

KAREN VOIGHT

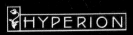
HYPERION

New York

The health, fitness, and nutritional information contained in this book is not intended to be a substitute for medical advice. Consult your physician before starting this or any other fitness program.

Art Direction & Design: Clifford Selbert Design Collaborative, Santa Monica

Library of Congress Cataloging-in-Publication Data

Voight, Karen, 1955–
        Voight: precision training for body and mind/Karen Voight.—1st ed.
        p. cm.
        ISBN 0-7868-8159-3
        1. Physical fitness for women. 2. Physical fitness for women—Psychological aspects.
        3. Exercise for women. 4. Diet.
I. Title.
GV482.V65 1996
613.7'045—dc20

FIRST EDITION
10 9 8 7 6 5 4 3 2 1

ACKNOWLEDGEMENTS

Thank you to Bob Miller for giving me the opportunity to create this book and to Wendy Lefkon for believing in my vision of what an exercise book can be. A big thank you to Paul Batoon for his endless patience and persistence in working with me and encouraging me every step of the way. Thanks to Brian & Tracey Lane for their unlimited creativity and imagination in putting this book together. Thank you to Laura Dayton and Kim Gross for helping me put my thoughts and experiences into words. Finally a special thank you to Eleanor Richman for making this book possible.

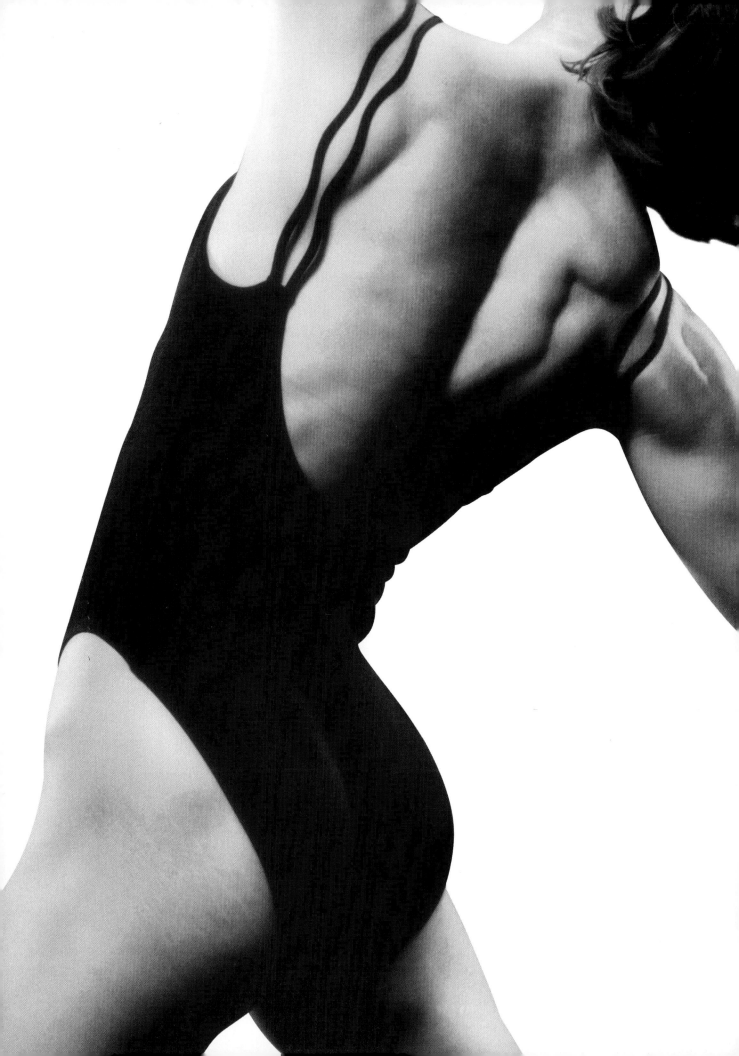

table of
CONTENTS

INTRO

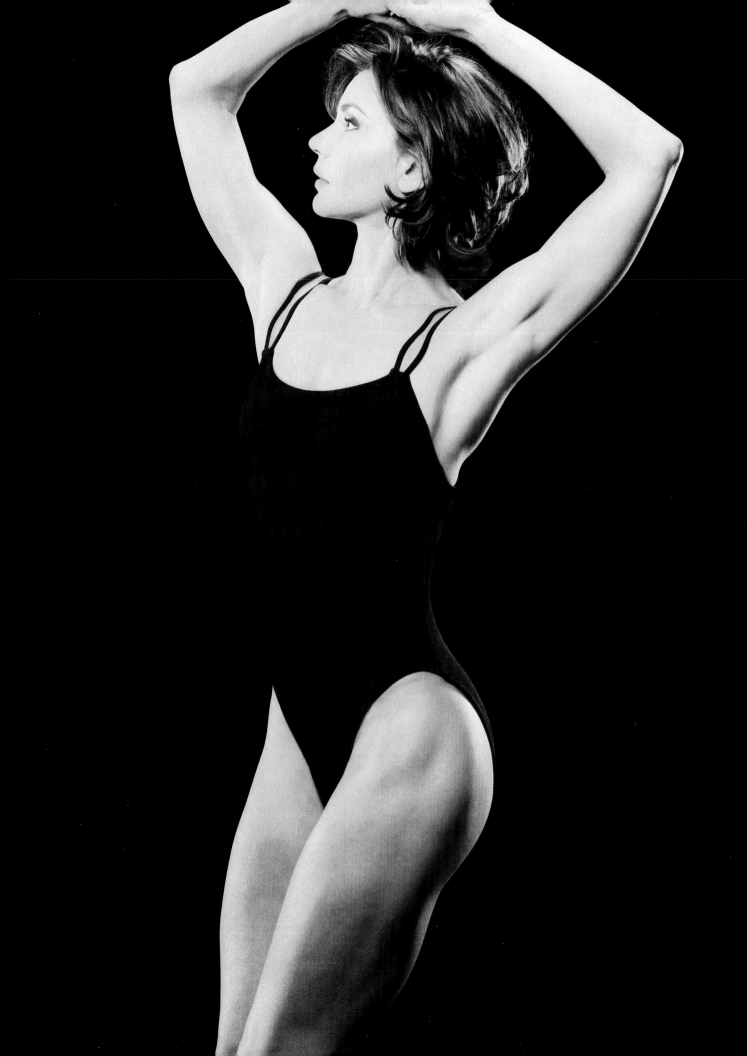

THIS IS AN EXERCISE BOOK Exercise is what I love and what I know best. For most of us, particularly women, exercise goals are nearly always directly tied to a goal of weight loss. So, while this is an exercise book, it is also a book about weight loss. Because fitness requires a body-mind approach, this book is about attitude, self-improvement and motivation.

Having watched thousands of individuals begin exercise programs, I've come to the conclusion that a synchronized approach, uniting body and mind, is the best way to achieve personal goals. Tackling exercise from a goal orientation, such as losing five pounds to fit into that bikini by summer, is valid in the short term — it provides an attainable target. But long-term results require a long-term commitment.

The core of this commitment is a complete understanding of the exercise process. This means becoming intimate with your body and tuning in to both the obvious and the subtle benefits of a healthy lifestyle. When this happens, exercise no longer becomes a dreaded task, but becomes as natural a part of daily life as showering, brushing your teeth, and getting dressed.

My role in your exercise program is to bring you the traditional elements of exercise — the exercises, sets, reps, tempo, intensity, and frequency — in a new context, with fresh information and insights. When exercise becomes one-dimensional and repetitive, even trainers become bored with their fitness programs.

I will encourage you to participate in the process of exercise and to develop a mind-set that will motivate you to commit to a fitness program. A biomechanically precise workout will be offered to help you accomplish your goals in the comfort of your home. I will also answer questions you have about how diet, age, and genetics affect the shape you're in, and about how these factors must all be considered when establishing your exercise goals.

STRAIGHT TALK Another part of my role is to help you wade through the confusing — and sometimes contradictory — information about fitness and nutrition so you can begin and stick with the program that is best for you. For years we were told that losing weight was a simple matter of cutting calories. Then we were told to forget counting calories because our bodies automatically revert to a set weight point. And then we learned that many people are born with a fat gene preprogrammed in their DNA.

Dietitians used to recommend eating pasta to lose weight. The same dietitians now declare that pasta is so calorically heavy it makes us fat. When it comes to exercise equipment, we pulled against resistance bands, then tossed them into the back of the closet alongside the gravity boots and rebounder — just in time to reach for the step and the slide.

Obviously, much of the information we receive is dictated not by what will really help us reach our exercise goals, but by what will boost a particular product's sales. My aim is to bring you real facts and real answers in a concise approach that is easy to understand and easy to put into action.

NEW TECHNOLOGY: OLD-FASHIONED BODIES Three components remain crucial to creating and maintaining a fit body: precision, perseverance, and patience. Unfortunately, in today's society we have little respect for patience. Even overnight delivery seems archaic when we can press a button and instantly fax or modem information. We live in a world where we crave immediate results. Here's the catch — the body is old-fashioned. There are no "magic" buttons and no overnight successes. Fitness takes time. To complicate matters, we have also imposed a much stricter image of what we want our bodies to look like. In many cases this image is not only unrealistic, it is unhealthy.

The truth is, it takes an extended length of time and concerted effort to achieve a fit and healthful body. Even though many of us spend enormous amounts of money trying to prove otherwise, there are no instant fixes. It is time to "bite the bullet," accept certain facts about your health and genetic potential, and approach your program in the most efficient and effective way possible.

Exercise is not always fun. It can be hard work, and it can sometimes be monotonous. If you assume that every workout will result in an endorphin-euphoria, you are setting yourself up for disillusionment and you will likely abandon your program. To succeed, exercise must be embraced as part of your lifestyle — not just an occasional, exhilarating rush. You will, at times, need to push yourself. But it will always pay off — and the payoff is evidenced not only by pride in accomplishment, but by a priceless increase in self-confidence and a renewed passion for life. Just as I've done in my videos, in this book I will illustrate how variety keeps a program interesting. I'll share motivational techniques that really work and provide you with precision moves that substantially increase your exercise skills. As you develop advanced skills, you will want to exercise more and you will elicit dramatic results — results that will prove to be the greatest motivator of all. My goal is to inspire you to develop a new perspective on exercise, one that makes it a priority in your life and keeps it in your life, for life.

WHAT it takes

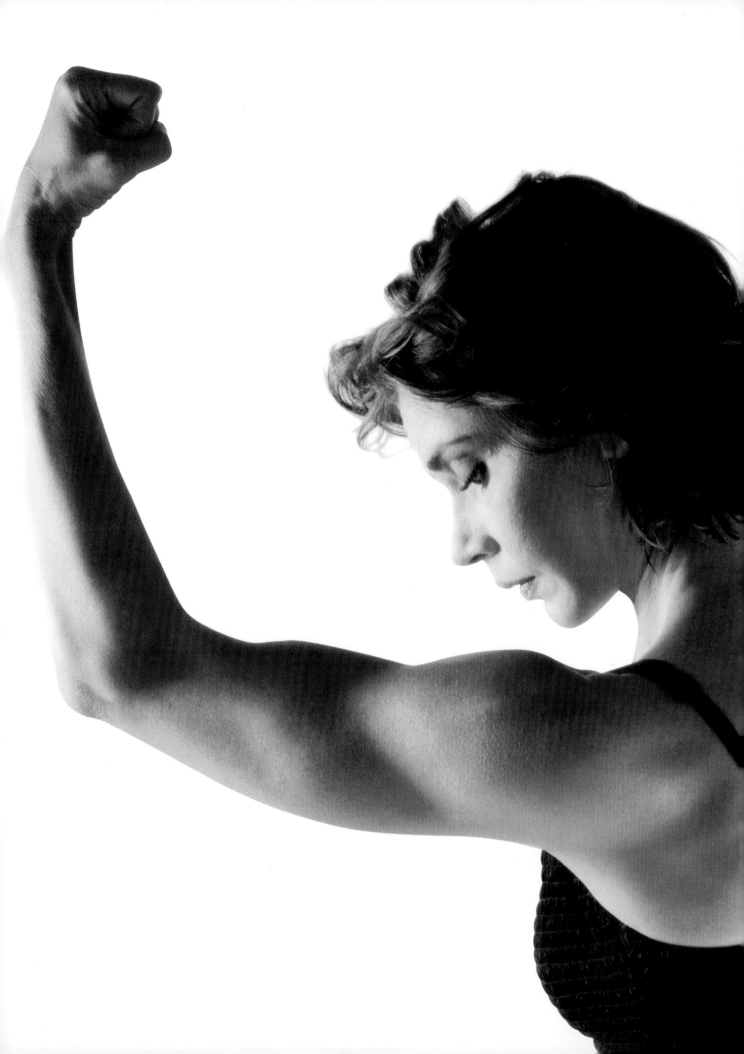

ANY TYPE OF PHYSICAL ACTIVITY—whether walking through a shopping mall or lifting heavy weights—is always beneficial. That's the beauty of a body in motion. The reason many people do not enjoy the benefits of regular exercise—including preventing illness—boils down to the tragic fact that most people just don't do it.

What separates those who achieve their "dream body" through exercise from those who do not has less to do with time and more to do with attitude. Developing an attitude that works for you is an individualized process. People who have succeeded in doing just that can be great motivators, and nowhere have I experienced a group of achievers more positive and driven than those I've encountered among Hollywood's elite.

I've personally trained many celebrities and have watched many more participate in my classes. Naturally, because of what they do, they are extremely motivated—they are in the public eye, and their progress is constantly monitored. Their physical attributes—hair, skin tone, every ounce of fat they gain or lose—is subject to intense scrutiny. They are *onstage* at all times, therefore they find it easier—in fact necessary—to immerse themselves frequently in a fitness routine. Celebrities present us with a marvelous example of how effort and the ability to focus on the task at hand can produce results. Here are some examples of the positive attitudes I've encountered in my classes and personal instruction.

BETTE MIDLER

Bette's secret for success—fun. She exploits her natural playfulness in everything she does, especially exercise. Her enjoyment is contagious, and she seems to rely on the strength of her sense of humor to get her through even the most grueling workouts. With her mind-set, Bette always manages to have a good time.

DIAHANN CARROLL

Totally focused, totally disciplined. I've been working with her for more than eight years and I never cease to be amazed by the communication she has with her own body. Diahann taught me that exercise instruction involves more than telling a person *what* to do with their body—you must also explain to them what the exercise *feels* like. In working with Diahann I've learned to tell people things like "squeeze your buttocks like you would a sponge" to help them recognize the feeling inside the muscles that exercise creates.

JAMES TAYLOR
He has a special ability to translate what I say into body language — immediately. The first time he attended my class I didn't know who he was, but I noticed his ability to execute every move perfectly and precisely. When I said "shoulders back," his shoulders went back. When I said "squat to parallel, with knees over your toes," his body was perfectly aligned. He has developed a heightened body awareness that enables him to hear the information, digest it, and use it.

STEPHANIE POWERS
Stephanie lets you know that she has to work just as hard as the rest of us to stay in shape. She is extremely consistent and sensitive when it comes to her body — she doesn't try to kick as high or as quickly as others, but performs the exercises with intensity appropriate to her level. She doesn't compare herself to anyone else; she individualizes the exercise to get the most from it. One look at her body tells you this technique works.

PAULA ABDUL
Because Paula comes from a dance background, she expects a tremendous amount from her body. She is conditioned to dance at peak performance at all times. She didn't lack the moves or the motivation, but had to be coached to pace herself. Like so many high achievers, Paula immediately assimilates information and turns it into practical action. She is very inspiring.

ELLE MACPHERSON
Perhaps because modeling is often learned by observing, Elle has a unique approach to exercise. She learns by watching the moves first, then applying a mental picture to the physical movement. When a move confused her she would watch closely while I demonstrated it until she could develop her own style of execution. Elle has a marvelous capacity to not be distracted by what everyone else is doing and to find what fits her body and her personality. She makes the exercise hers, not the instructor's.

WHY PROGRAMS FAIL Exercise programs fail primarily because people don't follow through. They abandon their program because it doesn't fit into their lifestyle, because they aren't mentally prepared, and because they don't know the proper methods. Most individuals do not have faith in the end result—a healthier and more beautiful body—and cannot envision it or use it as daily motivation.

Working in the fitness field, I've seen hundreds of people begin a program and stick with it. Unfortunately, I've seen hundreds more fail. Without question, seeing your body change, adapt, and benefit from the program is the greatest source of motivation. Until that happens, you need tools.

Make certain that you explore the many exercise options available to you. Personal trainers work. You need to find an individual who is qualified, motivated, and, most important, someone to whom you can relate. When it comes to a personal fitness program, ideally you will be able to learn sufficient skills from a trainer that will enable you to continue your program on your own.

If a personal trainer isn't an option, consider a workout partner. The right partner—one who is serious about his or her workout, consistent, dependable, on-time, and working close to your

level of conditioning—can provide motivation to get you and keep you on a program. It's easy to skip a workout on your own; but when you know someone is waiting for you, you're far less likely to cop out. If you don't know someone who would be a good workout partner, ask members of your club or class. Many people, just like yourself, are looking for someone to share their quest for better health. Making a monetary commitment to exercise—paying an hourly wage to a trainer or signing a contract at a health club—motivates some people to stick to a program . If you've had a tough time getting started, consider jump-starting your program with this type of commitment. Aerobic classes are ideal for most people, but they may not fit into your schedule. Weight training can be effective, but you also need a program to meet your cardiovascular needs, weight management goals, and strength levels.

For many, the best program is one you can do at home. If you opt for in-home training, approach it systematically and just as seriously as if you were paying membership dues. Schedule a certain time of the day for your workouts. You also need to establish a certain place for your workouts—whether it's in front of a television, in a spare room, or in your living room. Setting aside an exercise area that you pass during your regular activities is a constant reminder that exercise is a part of your daily routine.

THE PRIORITY PRINCIPLE Understanding

that exercise needs to be a priority in your life is essential

to staying on a program. For most of us that motivation

must come from within, which means prioritizing exercise

on a daily basis.

1 REALIZE THERE'S NO WAY AROUND IT. To stay in shape, lower body fat, and feel your best, you must exercise. Good intentions are not enough, nobody can do it for you, and if you don't do it then it's not going to get done. When you're tempted to stop and pick up the dry cleaning and forgo your exercise class, ask yourself whether the laundry can be squeezed into another part of the day, or if you're using this errand as an excuse. Clothes can only help you look good, but the exercise will make you look and feel good.

2 BROADEN YOUR RANGE OF ACTIVITIES. Having more choices of enjoyable activities that act as workouts will keep your exercise convenient. Put in the necessary planning so you're ready to go at a moment's notice. For example, because exercise is my livelihood, I keep a wide array of exercise resources so I can work out whenever the opportunity arises. If I'm not teaching a class one day, I can go to the local gym where I can use the treadmill, StairMaster,™ and weight equipment. If driving to the gym is not practical that day, I know of a route to take my dogs for a brisk walk that takes about 30 minutes. I've also devised a workout in the pool that includes 15 minutes of laps, followed by underwater squat jumps. I keep a file of current newsletters from the local hiking and biking clubs, so if I feel like it, I can join in. When traveling, I pack a jump rope and a Walkman with music tapes I've recorded ahead of time. The tapes have 45 minutes of nonstop music that I like, with a beat I can exercise to. My favorite activity to do on a rainy day is to choose a workout from my library of videotapes that not only energizes me, but also sparks my imagination to create my own new moves. On days where I want to do something physical, but not too strenuous, stretch and yoga classes are ideal. The best

trick I have is to keep a pair of tennis shoes and some shorts in the trunk of my car, so if I'm with a friend and have the chance to exercise, I don't have to go home to get my workout gear first.

3 REALIZE THAT TO KEEP EXERCISE A PART OF YOUR LIFE MAY REQUIRE REORGANIZATION AND CREATIVE JUGGLING. What works for me is to think of the amount of time I dedicate to exercise in terms of weekly blocks. For example, rather than tell myself I have to work out on Monday, Wednesday, and Friday, I would make a commitment to work out three times that week. This gives me more flexibility to be spontaneous with last-minute appointments, and it becomes a game to see how I can keep exercise high on the list without jeopardizing my other priorities. This technique is excellent for people with unpredictable schedules.

4 CREATE YOUR OWN SUPPORT SYSTEM. Socialize with those who understand your fitness goals and have a personal interest in exercise. You can exchange a lot of practical knowledge and useful information by sharing experiences with each other. Encourage friends and family to keep their eyes and ears open for any information that could help you achieve your goals. Many times I've discovered interesting books and articles this way.

EFFORT EQUALS RESULTS Every exercise program requires effort. It can be fun, exhilarating, and extremely satisfying, but it still requires effort. Frequently when I work out, the music and my body are in such perfect synchronization that I lose track of time—an hour class goes by in what seems like minutes. Effort is not necessarily laborious.

People who achieve their exercise goals learn to access energy and have a genuine 100 percent commitment to their program. Effort, unfortunately, is subject to individual interpretation. Many individuals claim they've put in everything they've got. Hundreds of people tell me how frustrated they've become after putting in time and effort and getting no results. But the fact is these people put in time, but only about 70 or 80 percent of genuine effort. If they were putting in 100 percent, they would be getting the results they want.

Motivational experts are familiar with this "80 percent threshold." Most people have no basis to gauge the energy they're expending, and at 80 percent many think they're giving it all. I find that even though the last 20 percent is the most difficult to pull out, accessing that last bit of effort makes all the difference in the results you attain.

The extra burst of energy that comes from giving 100 percent will translate into more calories

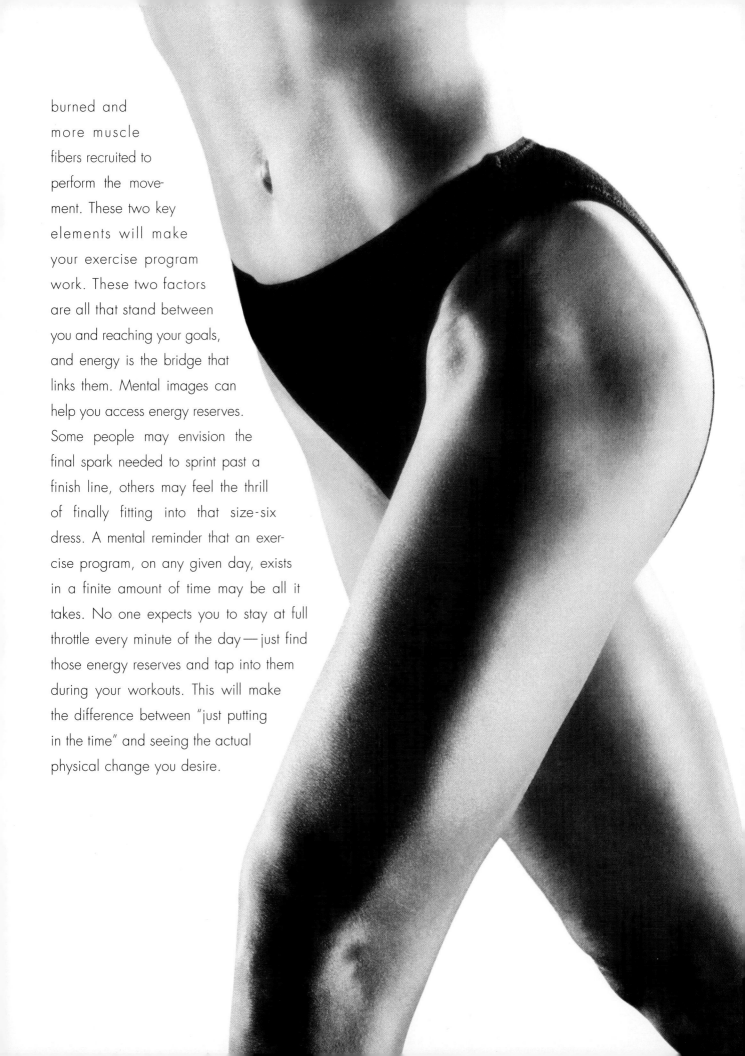

burned and
more muscle
fibers recruited to
perform the move-
ment. These two key
elements will make
your exercise program
work. These two factors
are all that stand between
you and reaching your goals,
and energy is the bridge that
links them. Mental images can
help you access energy reserves.
Some people may envision the
final spark needed to sprint past a
finish line, others may feel the thrill
of finally fitting into that size-six
dress. A mental reminder that an exercise program, on any given day, exists
in a finite amount of time may be all it
takes. No one expects you to stay at full
throttle every minute of the day — just find
those energy reserves and tap into them
during your workouts. This will make
the difference between "just putting
in the time" and seeing the actual
physical change you desire.

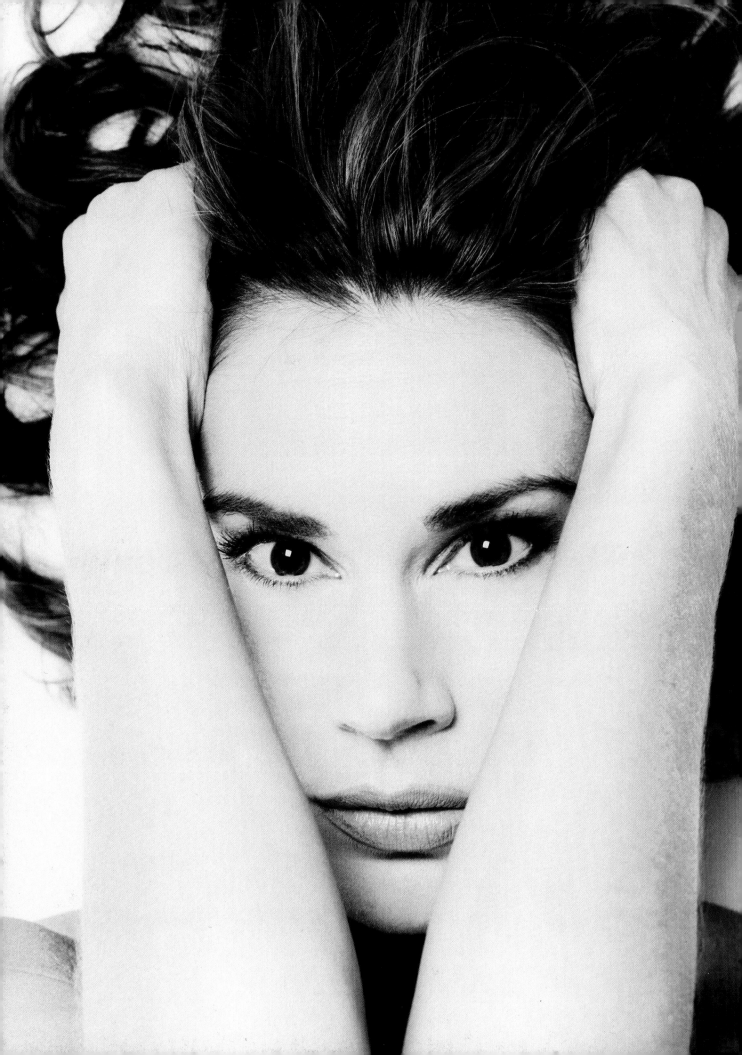

making up your MIND

WHILE I'VE LEARNED A GREAT DEAL from my celebrity clients, I've gained my most practical insights from working with individuals who are not in the public eye, and who have been able to find within themselves the motivation and energy to initiate a program, stick with it, and get the results they want.

I have observed common traits among individuals who succeed at their programs. The most critical of these traits is their mind-set toward exercising. Over the years, I've identified two distinct mind-sets: one is goal orientation, the other is process orientation. The key to success lies in understanding these two mental attitudes and interchanging them at the appropriate times. This mental agility — moving from goal to process — is what allows us to meet a challenge, initiate change, and stick with a program even during the inevitable plateaus we all experience.

GOAL VERSUS PROCESS Specific goals are what most often prompt someone to begin exercising. They have a high school reunion coming up and want to lose ten pounds in four weeks. They're headed for a beach house for the summer and want to look firm and toned in a swimsuit. Setting a goal is like creating a game plan — it gives us something to work toward. In time, however, that plan or goal — no matter how clearly defined at the beginning — fades from sight, especially when boredom creeps in.

That is when the second mind-set, *process*, comes into the picture. By relating to the process we find real satisfaction and genuine pleasure from the activity itself, rather than falling prey to boredom or discouragement. Using this state of mind, you'll focus on how good it feels. A process mind-set is particularly rewarding because it gives you a sense of empowerment, of taking control of your life and health. Setting goals gets you started but process orientation is what keeps you on track.

EVOLUTION OF EXERCISE MIND-SETS Not many exercise specialists acknowledge the existence of more than one mind-set. It's certainly easier to look just at goals. Goals are what get most Americans to work every morning. Initially, it can be a successful mind-set because it gets you going — but when it comes to exercise, just chasing a goal takes tremendous willpower and self-discipline and doesn't guarantee the person will continue, especially if she never enjoyed it in the first place.

For years, exercise was dominated by the goal-oriented mind-set. Looking back at those early days when women were becoming more serious about working out, I found they wanted a form of exercise that did more than accomplish a goal — they wanted to enjoy themselves in the process. What attracted them to my classes was a form of exercise that had rhythm, music, tempo, emotion and its own social climate. That is, of course, aerobic dance — a concept that caught on so quickly that few of us ever give a thought to the fact that just 20 years ago, the average person thought the word "aerobic" had something to do with flying.

Through my research on the effects of aerobic activity on women's bodies, I realized that duration of exercise was the key to raising metabolism and burning fat. So I began to incorporate 30- to 40-minute cardio segments during my classes — a brand-new concept at the time. My immediate challenge was to keep my students interested enough so they could actually enjoy these lengthy aerobic segments day after day. I wanted them to forget about time and be so totally absorbed in the activity that before they knew it, time was up. That was when I first identified the process-oriented mind-set as the key to helping them persist to achieve results.

This process-oriented mind-set can help you stick with any exercise program, whether it's aerobic dance, cycling, or floor exercises. You need to become immersed in the activity, both physically and mentally. Your success will be magnified when you get in touch with your body.

My style of exercise requires you to master a skill, which commands your attention and holds your interest in the "process." As you progress you will begin to anticipate and actually look forward to using those newly found skills in your next workout. "Getting it right" feels good and inspires you to want to do more. This attitude is the key to staying motivated.

Successful exercisers switch back and forth between mind-sets, although they probably don't realize it. Focus on goals and results whenever possible. But when you hit a dry spell and find yourself debating whether you want to work out on a given day, think about the process — how exercise makes you feel. Think about your body five minutes into a workout, when your muscles begin to warm and respond. Think of the invigorating feel of working up a good sweat. Remind yourself of the camaraderie and humor that is shared among other exercisers. Focus on the challenge of the exercise, how confident it makes you feel. Appreciate the escape that exercise provides — if you exercise by yourself this can actually be a time for mental as well as physical rejuvenation.

None of us has the luxury of remaining fit without working out. So go ahead and set your short-term goals and get satisfaction from meeting each one. Realize, however, that your greatest success will come when exercise fits naturally into your daily life and when you're able to gain genuine pleasure from just doing it.

getting
LEAN

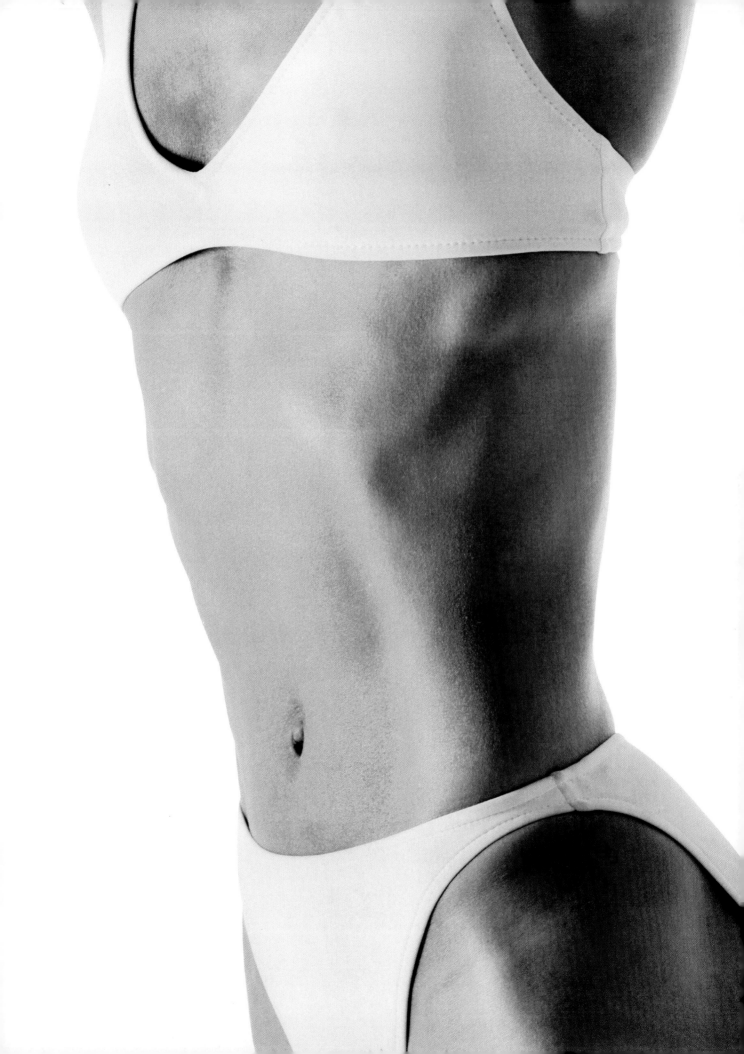

A LEAN BODY is attained through diet, exercise, and the proper attitude. This simple formula becomes complex when people confuse weight management — maintaining a healthy ratio of body fat and lean muscle — with trying to achieve the "ideal" body.

On magazine covers, in motion pictures, and on television shows we are confronted with a body image that is nearly impossible to achieve. This image is often the result of genetic luck, plastic surgery, or even photo retouching. The reality is that the average woman is 5 feet 4½ inches tall and weighs 140 pounds; however, the average model is 5 feet 10½ inches tall and weighs 117 pounds. A Barbie doll in real life would measure 39-18-33 and would topple head-over-toes if she tried to walk! Even the measurements of mannequins have shrunk over the past 40 years.

These unreal body images have made weight loss an endless struggle. Some people, in their blind ambition to emulate this unreal ideal, have resorted to extremely unhealthy behaviors. Their exercise becomes compulsive, literally eclipsing other aspects of their life, or they become afflicted with life-threatening eating disorders such as anorexia and bulimia.

There is a middle ground. Without going to extremes, it is possible to adjust diet, curb food cravings, exercise on a regular basis, and achieve a body shape that is attractive and in accordance with a person's genetic potential. That's realistic; and that's where I'm coming from.

WOMEN AND WEIGHT LOSS Managing body weight is a problem for both men and women, but many factors make weight control more difficult for women. Fat storage has been programmed into the female genetic code. Women have a difficult time losing weight because we are biologically designed to bear children. Our reproductive organs require a certain amount of body fat to function — when body fat drops below this minimum, menstrual cycles temporarily stop. A woman's body is also programmed to store fat efficiently. This is to protect a developing fetus from being denied nutrients, a biological function that was extremely important when famines were common. The female body is prepared to store enough fat for the fetus to grow for nine months, even when the crops fail. Only in the past half-century has there been no serious threat of famine, and there is simply no way to convince genetic programming that the threat has passed.

Women also burn fat in a highly efficient manner. To protect precious fat stores, women take longer to begin optimally burning fat, about 20 minutes into exercise. They also stop burning fat sooner than men, about an hour after exercise. Men, on the other hand, may start burning fat as soon as they begin exercising and continue for hours after exercise.

These biological differences in how the sexes store and use fat mean that two people can live under the same roof, eat the same foods, jog together on the same days, and basically expend equal effort performing day-to-day activities, but the man may remain lean while the woman gains weight. How many women have felt they'd failed when their husbands could control their weight but they could not? How many husbands looked at their wives as though they were weak-willed, chocolate-hoarding failures? Certainly, these false assumptions have led to needless self-criticism and unhappiness for many people. Yet the psychological ramifications extend beyond those imposed by our biology; women also think differently about food than men.

Food is not only a source of enjoyment for most women but a part of our basic nature. Women are the nurturers of the species; our involvement with food is intrinsically linked to family and friends. For women, the attitude that weight loss can *only* be accomplished by restricting food carries many negative repercussions. By denying themselves food many women become prisoners of their bodies. The result has been internal psychological conflicts that have manifested themselves as anger, depression, compulsive behavior, and eating disorders.

Fortunately, we now know that weight management is not just a matter of restricting food but also requires changing eating habits and adding a regular program of exercise. This combination will bring control over our weight within our reach.

EXERCISE, DIET, AND WEIGHT LOSS Exercise is necessary to get the weight off—and absolutely essential to *keep* it off. In addition to burning calories, most physical activities contribute to weight management by increasing or maintaining lean muscle tissue. Different types of tissue require different amounts of energy for sustenance. It should come as no surprise that fat sits on your body and requires very few calories. Muscle, on the other hand, is a vital and active tissue that is constantly burning calories, even while at rest.

The amount of lean muscle tissue you have is key to controlling your weight. You need to build it and then maintain it. This is the only way to increase your metabolism, thereby allowing you to eat satisfying meals, while keeping your weight under control.

Developing muscle mass does not mean that you will need to develop the figure of a bodybuilder. Certain types of exercise contribute more to muscle mass than others. Strength training moves are the best, but resistance should always be light to moderate so you don't overdevelop the muscle. Performing movements that use many large muscles together, such as squatting or lunging, also helps to build muscle mass without the bulkiness associated with bodybuilding.

WHAT'S REAL FOR YOU Weight loss goals must be established with a sensible assessment of what you can realistically accomplish for yourself. If you have a blocky build and a thick waist, you can sculpt a lean, athletic figure but you will never achieve the waiflike proportions of some of today's 90-pound, 5-foot-6-inch models. It is helpful to look through the magazines and media for other people with similar body types and examine what they've accomplished.

If you are short with a small frame, look at some of the changes Madonna and Janet Jackson have accomplished. If you are tall with a large frame, look at Linda Carter and Gabrielle Reece as examples of what you can do. When you've found the image you want—fit, lean, and firm— use it as your guide, but be certain the person is similar to you in height, build, bone density, age, and fat-accumulation sites. Many people cut out photos and use them for motivation.

If you have battled a weight problem your entire life, don't expect things to change overnight. Studies have shown that continual dieting that results in weight lost and weight regained may make your ultimate weight loss more difficult.

Continually dieting to lose weight without exercising affects muscle mass. With each successive diet, the body loses more muscle mass. Even if the dieter gains and loses the same 20 pounds, the ratio of fat to muscle in their body changes, and the fat percentage increases. As time goes on, the higher percentage of body fat causes the body to slow down and use fewer calories for energy. Thus, even though the dieter is eating the same amount of food, more of it is now turning to fat. The end result is the dieter continues to gain back more fat weight with each successive diet.

The good news is that an exercise program can stop the rebound effect. By building back the lean muscle tissue, the body's metabolism will change, although it may take your body months or even a year to begin efficiently using calories again.

A LIFESTYLE APPROACH Some lucky individuals go through their entire lives never having to worry about weight management. They are rare exceptions. Even those who manage to skate through their twenties and thirties may find weight a formidable opponent as they get older. This is true in both men and women; but as women reach their menopausal years, hormonal changes affect their weight-gain patterns and they experience a shift from weight accumulating in their hips, thighs, and buttocks, to their upper body, back, and waist. It seems like a battle that can't be won. For all of us, getting older means eating less and exercising more. Accepting this as a fact of life is the first and most important step to a healthy attitude.

The latest statistics estimate that almost one-third of Americans are overweight. Is this any surprise, considering our access to high-fat foods, and our sedentary lifestyle? Many Europeans still rely on walking and bicycling to get around for daily chores, and statistically European populations have lower percentages of body fat. How many Americans even consider walking a half mile to the grocery store, let alone do it?

I don't expect you to toss the car keys, but you need to realize that movement—daily movement—is essential to weight management, and without it, the odds are that you are going to get fat. You need to learn to keep your energy up,

all day. Putting extra effort into exercise burns more calories, and putting extra energy into every activity in your life increases the calories you burn as well.

CALORIES EXPENDED If you need to lose weight it is essential to begin performing activities that are fat-burning in nature. It's important to recognize that prolonged aerobic activity isn't the only way to burn fat calories. Intense, short-burst activities, such as tennis or strength training in the gym, cause the body to release a chemical called noradrenaline. This chemical is a powerful fat-burner, and while the activity may not be continuous enough to cause your body to go after its fat stores, the release of noradrenaline will cause your body to utilize more fat for energy following the workout.

CREATIVE CALORIE BURNERS It doesn't matter whether it's walking up the stairs instead of taking the escalator or carrying all the grocery bags in yourself instead of asking for help, you need to look at your life for opportunities to expend more energy and burn more calories. Be creative in making everyday activities a form of exercise.

Many years ago when I was modeling in a swimwear studio, I found myself in the predicament of spending long hours waiting for appointments. I was stuck in a room and getting no exercise, yet I was supposed to look perfect. I solved the problem by volunteering to get everyone's coffee—knowing the café was up 13 flights of stairs! Three or four times a day I would climb those 13 flights for a great step workout.

At another point in my early career I was working in downtown Los Angeles and found myself with the same dilemma of not being able to fit in my workouts. There was a rather expensive parking lot in the basement of my building. I had to be at work at 8 A.M. and could have easily used the basement lot. Instead, I found a parking lot nearly three-quarters of a mile away. Not only was it less expensive, but it served as my morning workout. I pulled into the lot at 7:40 A.M., changed to my tennis shoes, and walked to work at a fast pace.

While I don't fetch coffee anymore, I still search out parking spaces at the furthest reasonable distance from the door. I've also found that in my office, placing the file cabinet in a corner away from my desk gets me out of my chair more often. By putting my most referenced papers in the bottom drawer, my legs, thighs, and butt get even more attention from the additional bending. Instead of constantly looking for ways to avoid extra activity, I purposely create these little "inconveniences" each day and see them as bonus muscle-movers with "fitness dividends." They add up at the end of the week so I can look back and congratulate myself on having so creatively cheated nature out of storing an extra ounce of fat on my body.

There are hundreds of ways you can add to your bonus exercise time. Have household chores to perform? Do them with extended movements as quickly as possible to reap the most exercise benefit. When an appointment gets canceled, look at this as a chance to get in an extra workout.

Wear comfortable shoes and nonrestrictive clothes whenever possible. Ever notice when you're wearing a tight skirt and high heels that your physical activity is severely limited? A simple way to increase the activity you do is to dress properly. I try to wear comfortable, stretch clothing and flat shoes every chance I can. Dressing this way encourages me to be energetic and on the move. Every incremental bit of exercise adds up—you don't need to get all your exercise in at one 20- or 30-minute session. Five minutes here and there all add up to keep fat at bay.

Begin making physical activities such as dancing, walking, hiking, scuba diving, bicycling, skiing, skating, golf, or tennis part of your life. There are literally hundreds of activities to get involved in, and even if you do one or two just once a month, you will burn more calories.

By using every opportunity to get up and move, you can win half the battle of controlling your weight. And of course, the more calories you burn, the less you will need to restrict what you eat.

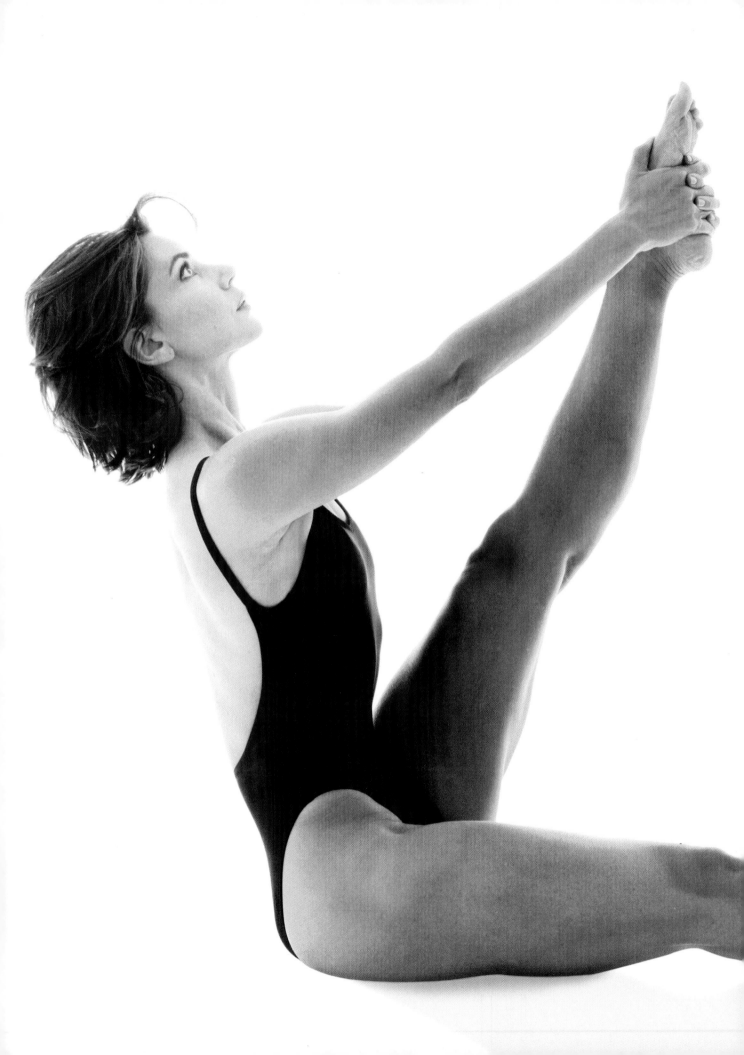

precision

PAYS OFF

A SIMPLE WAY to determine what a particular exercise program can do for you is to look at the body of an individual who follows that program. If you want to look like a runner, train like a runner. If you want to look like a weightlifter, eat and work out like one. If you want to look like a dancer, perform a dancer's movements.

My workouts are designed to refine the body: to lower body fat and bring out muscular definition, not to develop thick, large muscles. I use exercises to increase functional strength, cardiovascular fitness, and overall good health. The exercises in this book develop muscular strength and endurance similar to that of a dancer or an endurance athlete such as a cyclist or distance runner.

I've created routines for you to do on your own in your home. They rely on focused movements — some of them require only your body weight, others use light weights for resistance. These exercises are strategically arranged to work each body region in a compound fashion that warms up your muscles. Then I target specific muscles for individual attention. These exercises should be performed consistently and will be the basis of your strength-training and muscle-sculpting work. By engaging in regular aerobic activity like biking, walking, stair climbing, or aerobic dance, you will have all the tools to achieve your desired body shape.

THE FIVE FACTORS Five guidelines must be followed to achieve low body fat and defined muscles, particularly in women. These are:

1 MODERATE INTENSITY – perform exercises at approximately 70 to 75 percent of your maximum strength.

2 HIGH FREQUENCY – exercise on a consistent, four-, five- or six-day per week schedule, depending on your ability and conditioning level.

3 LONG DURATION – use maximum repetitions, until your muscles are fatigued.

4 LOWER BODY EMPHASIS – perform more exercises for your legs, hips, and buttocks than for your upper body.

5 COMPOUND FOLLOWED BY AN INDIVIDUAL EXERCISE – always begin with a movement that works several muscles before performing an exercise that targets a single one.

MODERATE INTENSITY allows you to train almost daily and will avoid overtraining. Overtraining, which manifests itself in sore muscles, chronic fatigue, and a susceptibility to illness, occurs when you exercise at your maximum strength threshold on a daily basis. This overtraining syndrome is not to be confused with applying 100 percent effort in your exercise. Remember that 100 percent effort requires concentration on technique and can be done at a moderate intensity. Allow your muscles to fatigue, and when you feel you cannot complete more than three to five more repetitions, stop. That represents your 70 to 75 percent threshold.

HIGH FREQUENCY and LONGER DURATION allow the muscles to get stronger without building size. A bodybuilder who wants to create size purposely trains for brief, very intense periods, followed by rest days so that the muscle can grow. Exercising for longer durations on a daily or high-frequency basis ensures different results. The exercises in this book develop muscular endurance by training the muscles through a prolonged period of time.

STRESSING THE LOWER BODY is a relatively new concept in exercise philosophies. Many women are joining health clubs and gyms, only to find that most of the equipment is geared toward upper body work, which appeals primarily to men. Some male personal trainers persist in coaching women with strength routines that I think would be better suited to a man's body. I have heard this frustration expressed to me time and again by my female clients. Aerobic classes come closer to addressing the needs of a woman's body. It is a fact that most women are interested in decreasing the size of the hips, thighs, waist, and buttocks, and don't really care about the circumference of their biceps. The key to lower-body slimming is frequent lower body work with light resistance and heavy repetitions.

Each of my body part routines relies on a system of COMPOUND MOVEMENTS FOLLOWED BY INDIVIDUAL MUSCLE WORK. This means that I begin each of my body part routines with exercises that simultaneously recruit several muscle groups at once, and follow up with exercises to target the individual muscle. In this way the individual muscle is sufficiently fatigued without having to work at maximum strength loads. This keeps the muscle from developing bulk and size.

WHEN SORENESS IS OK When performing exercises for any muscle group, you may experience some muscle soreness. This is normal and is a response of the muscle adapting to the work load.

Primary muscle soreness usually occurs within a few hours of exercise and peaks in about 24 hours. While it can sometimes be uncomfortable, there are no long-lasting effects from this type of soreness. If it occurs, warm baths or saunas help, as will stretching and light massage. If the muscle soreness is severe, skip a day or two of exercise until it subsides. Each subsequent workout will produce less and less muscular soreness, until you reach a point where the soreness is just a pleasant reminder that your program is working. There are various sensations you'll experience in your muscles when you exercise. A feeling of heat in the muscle refers to a condition that occurs after a long duration of exercise, such as after your last set or repetition. It is caused by a build-up of lactic acid within the muscle and will subside as soon as you stop the movement. This feeling is often felt in muscle groups that respond well to long duration exercise — the abdominals, the calves, and sometimes the legs.

Your muscles may often feel fatigue. This feeling is quite different from exhaustion and is a signal that you are reaching your 70 to 75 percent threshold. Fatigue is the point that ends any given set of exercise. I provide a system of repetitions and sets, but the savvy exerciser will adjust these according to her individual level of fatigue. Exhaustion, on the other hand, is usually accompanied by pain in the working muscle. It makes you unable to finish the amount of repetitions on a particular set and is a signal that you are working beyond the moderate intensity level of 70 to 75 percent.

BREATHING Proper breathing is an absolute necessity in your exercise program. Breathing carries essential nutrients to your working muscles. Your breathing is also an indicator of how hard your heart is working — never exercise to a point where you are unable to speak in a normal conversational tone. Breathing can help make exercise easier to perform. The general rule is to inhale at the start of the movement, exhale during the exertion.

This means when performing a squatting movement, inhale as you bend at the knees and lower, exhale as you push yourself back to the top of the movement. To help remind them to stay aware of their breathing, many people practice exhaling through their mouth so they actually hear themselves breathing in a slow, controlled, and constant manner throughout their workout.

PATIENCE Lastly, have patience. If you are not accustomed to precision exercise you will need to learn, or perhaps relearn, these movements. Just as you can correct posture at any age, you can also teach your body to move in a more fluid way. Precise movement is acquired through practice and becomes more familiar through repetition. Don't allow yourself to give up too soon just because you lack the patience. Remember, practice makes perfect, and I'd like to add that precision pays off.

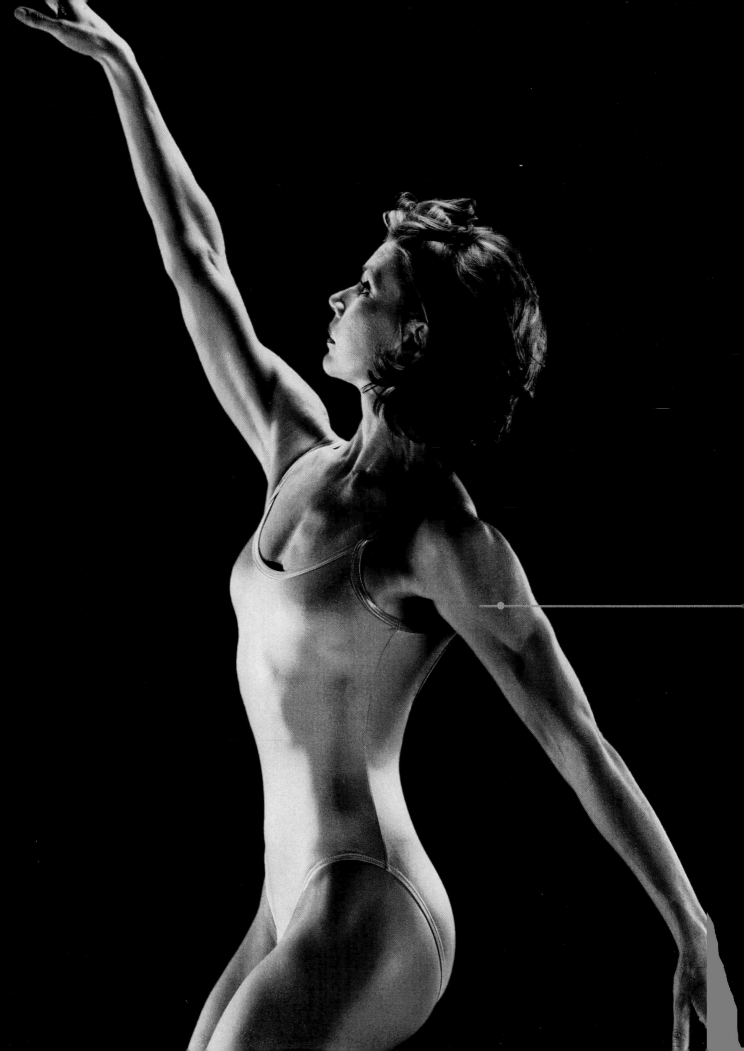

arms SCULPT

ARMS Upper body training imparts a graceful appearance to your arms and shoulders, and provides extra power for day-to-day activities that require lifting, pushing, and pulling. The exercises in this routine require integrated movement, recruiting the muscles not only in your arms, but your chest and shoulders.

In this way it serves as the foundation for a well-balanced upper body program. | Extra attention is placed on the tricep muscle which accounts for 70 percent of the muscle mass in your upper arm. Genetically, women tend to accumulate fat in this area and if neglected it becomes quite flabby. But what looks like fat is often just a lack of muscle tone and can be quickly shaped up. | I've chosen exercises that use a combination of your own body's resistance, light hand weights, and my 12-pound Voight Bar. I recommend using high repetitions and stress the importance of performing the exercises in the exact order they are presented. This is true in subsequent exercise chapters as well. | Perfect form is essential — the body often finds ways to cheat or perform less work. When using weights, do not rely on momentum by swinging the weight. | Begin with a light weight (1 to 2 pounds) then work up to heavier weights (3 to 4 pounds). Whether you're using weights or not, remember this key training tip: Always hold for a two-count beat at the top, and bottom, of every movement. Asserting this type of control in your training stimulates the deep muscle fibers and ensures maximum results from your efforts.

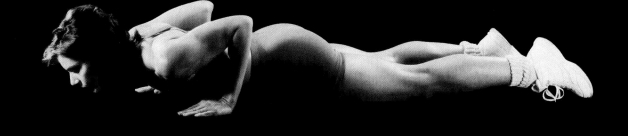

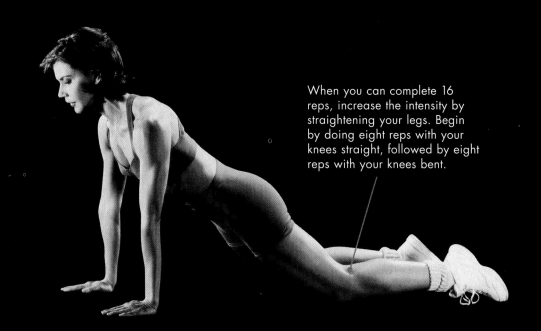

When you can complete 16 reps, increase the intensity by straightening your legs. Begin by doing eight reps with your knees straight, followed by eight reps with your knees bent.

push-up   *(chest, shoulders, triceps)*

(a) Lie face down and place your hands directly underneath your shoulders. Your fingers should face forward with your elbows tucked in and back. Keep your head in line with your spine — don't look up! Your back should be straight, with the abdominal muscles pulled in.

(b) Balancing on your knees, lift your upper body by pushing with your arms until they are straight. During this movement your elbows should point back rather than to the side. Pause at the top for two seconds and then slowly lower to the start. Repeat for 16 repetitions.

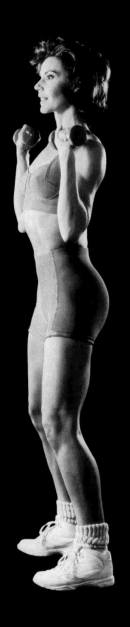

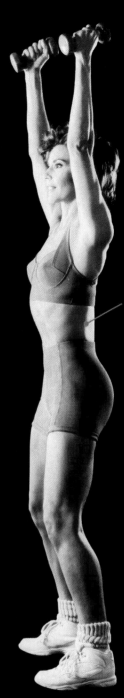

If you find yourself arching your back as you press the weights overhead, try performing the exercise with one leg forward and the other leg back, legs about 18 inches apart.

overhead press *(shoulders, triceps, upper back)*

a   Assume a standing position with your knees slightly bent and abdominal muscles pulled in. Hold the hand weights in front of your shoulders, palms facing away from your body.

b   Press the hand weights directly overhead, gradually rotating your arms so that your palms are facing each other at the top. Lower to the start position with palms facing out. Perform 16 repetitions.

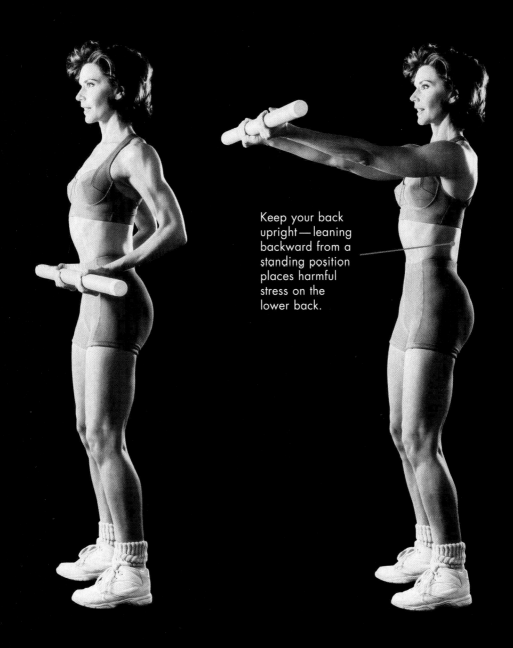

Keep your back upright—leaning backward from a standing position places harmful stress on the lower back.

scoop-outs *(front delts, biceps)*

ⓐ Grasp a 12-pound bar or hold two-to-five pound hand weights. Turn your palms up and spread your hands shoulder-width apart. Start with the bar at your hip bones with your elbows pointed back.

ⓑ "Scoop" your arms up and out until the bar is level with your shoulders, hold for two seconds, then slowly return to the start. Do 12 repetitions, working up to 16.

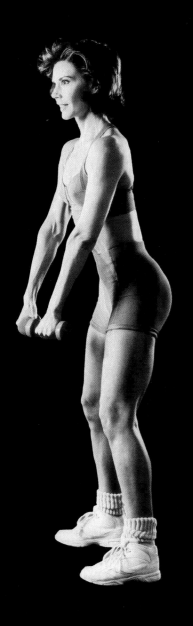
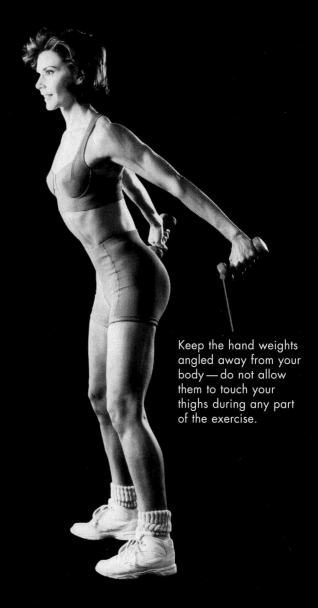

Keep the hand weights
angled away from your
body — do not allow
them to touch your
thighs during any part
of the exercise.

push backs *(rear delts, triceps)*

a Using two-to-five pound hand weights, stand with your feet shoulder-width apart and your knees slightly bent. Pull your lower abdominals in tight, and lean forward from the hips with shoulders in front of your knees. Hold the weights together in front of you, directly under your chin, with your palms facing you.

b Pull the weights back and out, fully squeezing your shoulder blades together at the finish. Hold this peak contraction for two seconds before returning to the start. Do 16 repetitions.

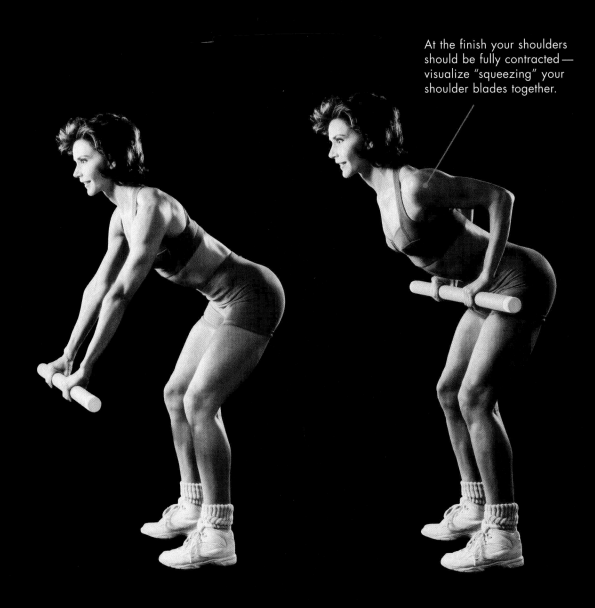

At the finish your shoulders should be fully contracted — visualize "squeezing" your shoulder blades together.

bent-over rows

(lats, rear delts, glutes, hamstrings, back extensors)

(a) Hold a bar or five-pound hand weights with your palms facing down, hands shoulder-width apart. Bend your knees slightly and lean forward from the hips so that your back forms a 45-degree angle to the floor. Keep your head in line with your back.

(b) Pull the bar to your navel, keeping your elbows tucked in and back and your chest lifted. Pause for two seconds at the top of the movement and then slowly return to the start. Perform 16 repetitions, working up to 24 reps.

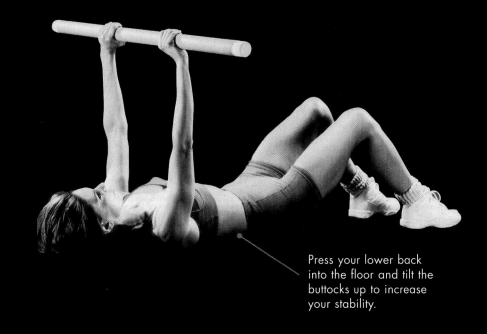

Press your lower back
into the floor and tilt the
buttocks up to increase
your stability.

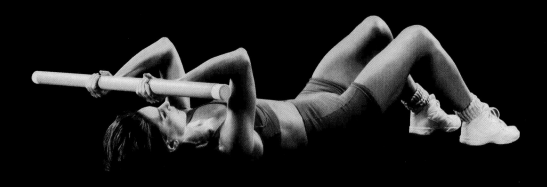

vertical extension *(triceps)*

a Lie on your back with your knees bent. Grasp a bar or two three-to-five-pound hand weights with a shoulder-width grip, palms facing forward. Press the weights up to straight arms.

b Keeping your upper arms perpendicular to the floor and elbows pointed toward your knees, slowly lower the weight to the top of your head, pause for two seconds, then press the weight back to the start position. Don't let your elbows flare out to the side as this can be harmful to the shoulders. Perform 16 repetitions, progressing to 24 reps.

STRONG legs

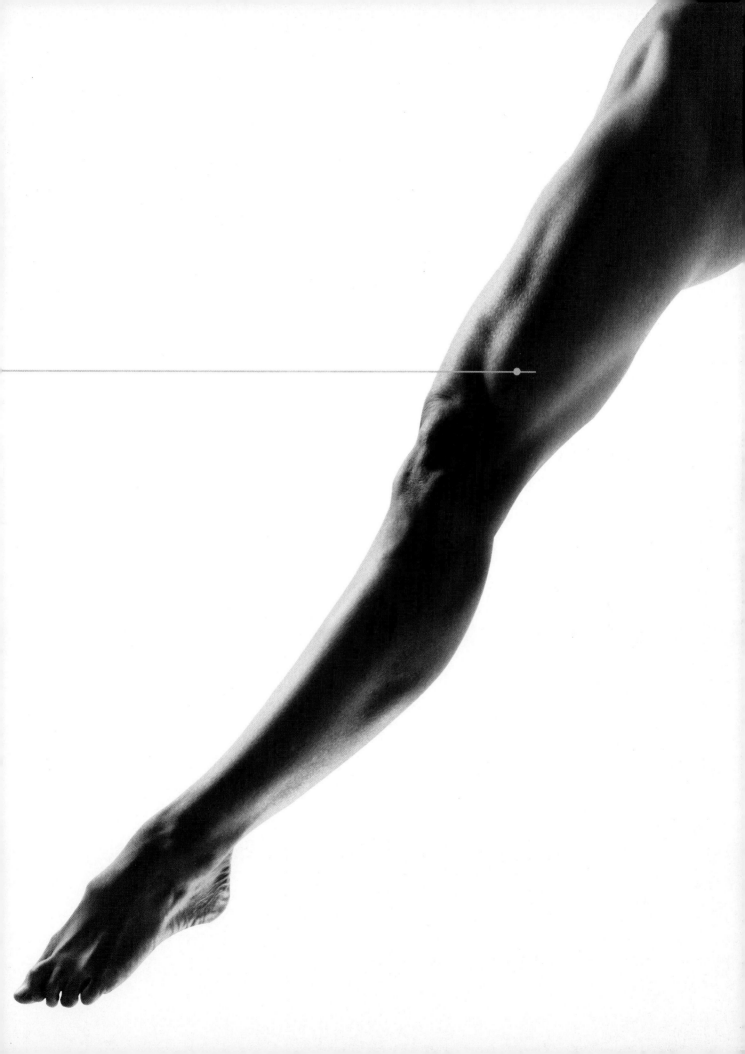

LEGS For most women, the lower body is the most difficult to keep fat-free and firm. Three areas of the leg present the toughest challenges. First is creating a distinct separation between the buttocks and the back of the leg. Next is the shaping of the front of the thigh, specifically the area just above the knee. The third problem area is the inner thigh. | This program addresses each of these. It also carries bonus benefits: not only do a pair of well-conditioned legs look sleek and sexy, but keep in mind that the extra effort you put into your leg training translates into extra calories burned and a decrease in overall body fat. Therefore, the more time spent in your routine working the lower body results in faster weight loss, a leaner physique, and greater satisfaction from your exercise program. | When the exercises in this routine are done regularly and precisely, your results are virtually guaranteed. Attention to detail will make the difference. Because all muscles work in teams, some of these movements will also incorporate the muscles of the buttocks. In the next chapter, when you work the buttocks, some of those movements will also require the muscles of the legs. This double-team approach to the lower body allows you to burn maximum calories in this workout, while providing maximum emphasis on toning and sculpting the lower body.

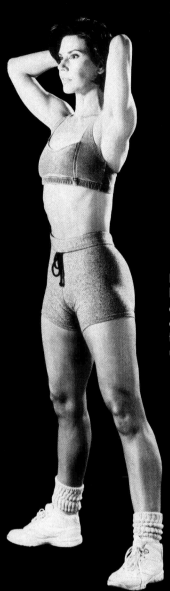

Place a 12-pound Voight bar on your shoulders for additional resistance. Also, do not let your chest fall forward as this causes the upper back to round.

toe out squats *(quadriceps, gluteals, hamstrings)*

(a) Stand with your feet slightly wider than shoulder-width, toes pointed just slightly out. Place your hands behind your head and pull the abdominal muscles in while lifting the chest.

(b) Squat down until your thighs are parallel to the floor, hips pressed behind heels. Hold this position for two seconds and then stand up. As you stand rotate your hips forward, squeezing your buttocks tight without locking your knees. Perform 16 to 24 repetitions.

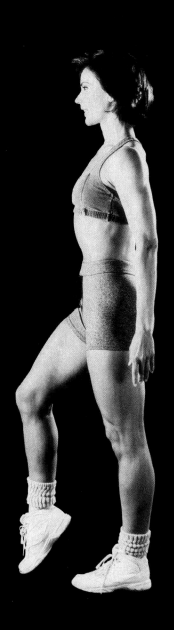

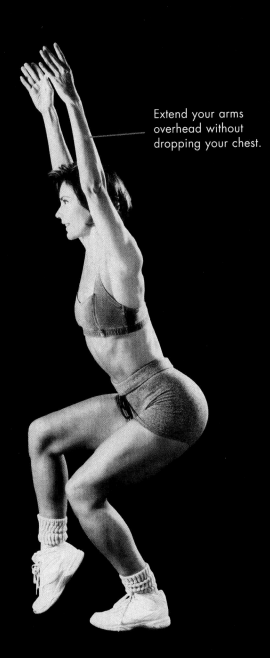

Extend your arms
overhead without
dropping your chest.

one-legged squats *(quadriceps, gluteals)*

(a) From a standing position, place your right foot about four to six inches in front of your left and let your hands rest at your sides.

(b) Shifting your balance so that the majority of your weight is on your rear foot, bend your knees until your front thigh is almost parallel to the floor. Pause for two seconds at the bottom of the squat, and then come out of the squat by rotating your hips forward and squeezing your buttocks.

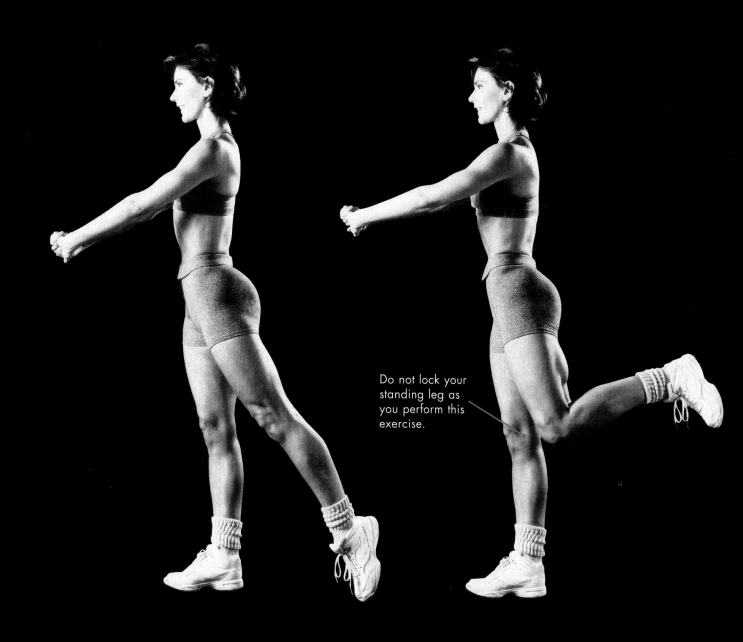

Do not lock your standing leg as you perform this exercise.

hamstring curls *(hamstrings)*

a From a standing position, place your left foot about 18 inches behind the right. Extend your arms in front of you for balance.

b Bring your left heel toward your glutes by squeezing the hamstring, keeping your left thigh stationary. Hold the top position for two seconds before returning your leg to the start. Keep your abdominal muscles pulled in to support your lower back. Do 16 repetitions and then switch to the other leg.

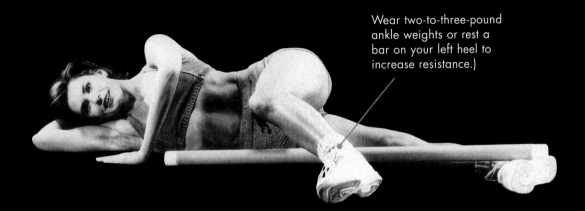

Wear two-to-three-pound ankle weights or rest a bar on your left heel to increase resistance.)

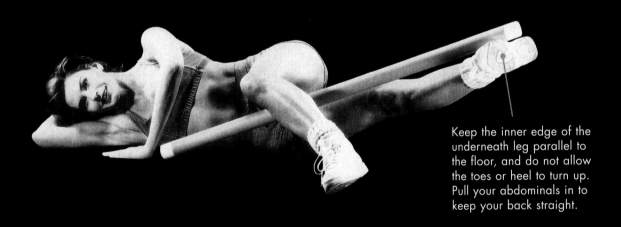

Keep the inner edge of the underneath leg parallel to the floor, and do not allow the toes or heel to turn up. Pull your abdominals in to keep your back straight.

inner thigh lifts   *(inner thigh)*

a Lie on your left side and fold your left arm under your neck to support your head. Straighten your left leg until your heel is in line with your shoulders. Cross the right leg over your left, bending the knee with your foot on the floor.

b Lift your left leg as high as you can, which should be about 8 to 12 inches, pause for two seconds, then slowly return to the start. Do 16 repetitions and work up to 24 with each leg.

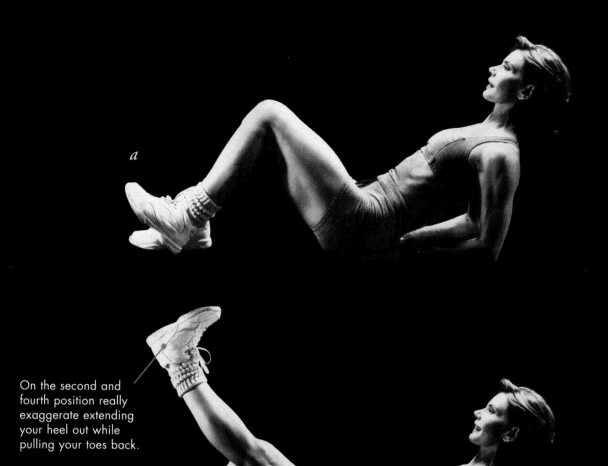

a

b

On the second and fourth position really exaggerate extending your heel out while pulling your toes back.

quad extensions *(quadriceps, calves)*

(*a*) In a sitting position, support yourself on your hips and elbows with your knees bent and one foot flat on the floor. Your other heel should rest on the floor.

(*b*) Keeping your knees at the same level, tense the front of your thigh and extend one leg out with a flexed foot.

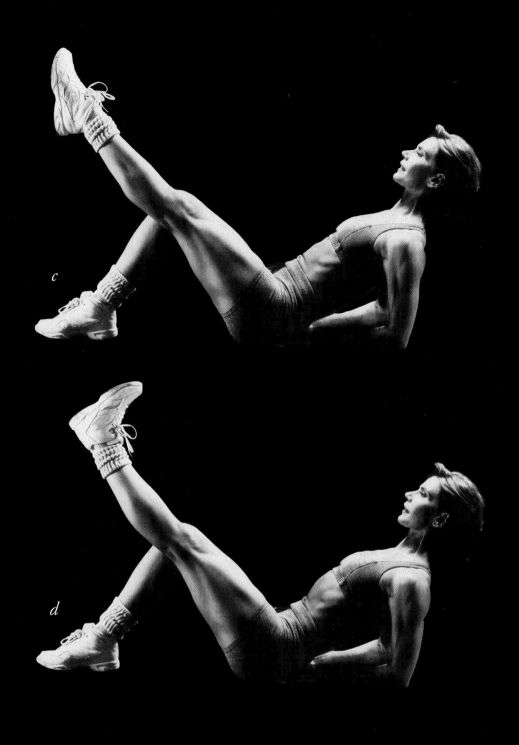

c Point your toes by squeezing your calf...

d ...then flex your foot again before returning to the start position.

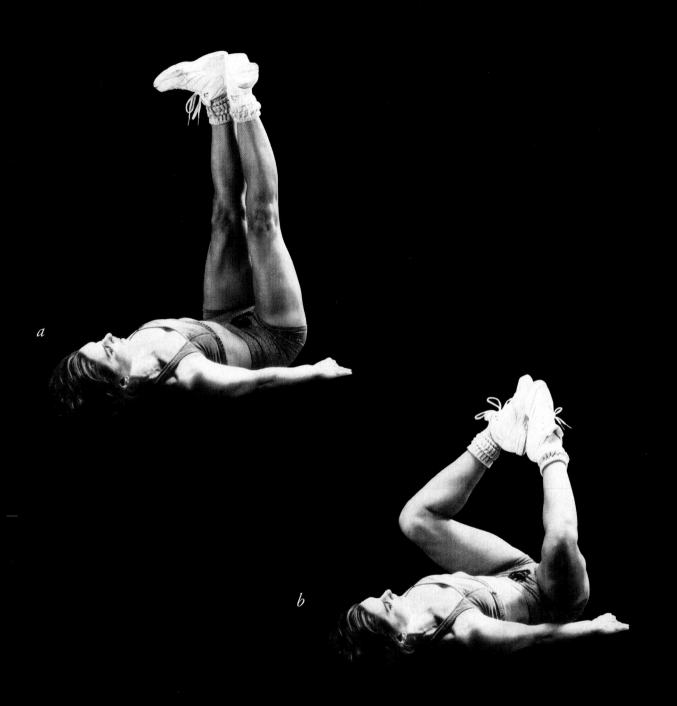

inner thigh squeeze-ins (inner thighs, sartoriu.

a Lie on your back with your hands at your sides. Extend your legs straight up until they are perpendicular to the floor. Rotate your legs out and with your heels together flex your feet.

b Point your toes and bend your knees, opening your knees outward.

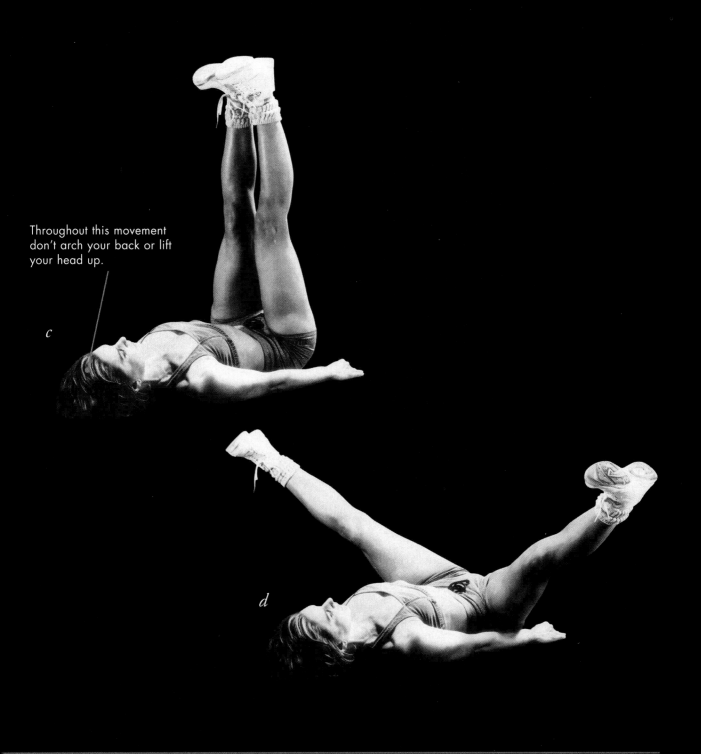

Throughout this movement don't arch your back or lift your head up.

c

d

(*c*) Push your legs up and straight. Flex your feet, turning them to a parallel position.

(*d*) Slowly split your legs apart while keeping them parallel. Pause for two seconds at the bottom, then slowly squeeze your legs back together in a parallel position. Do 16 repetitions and work up to 24.

FIRM buttocks

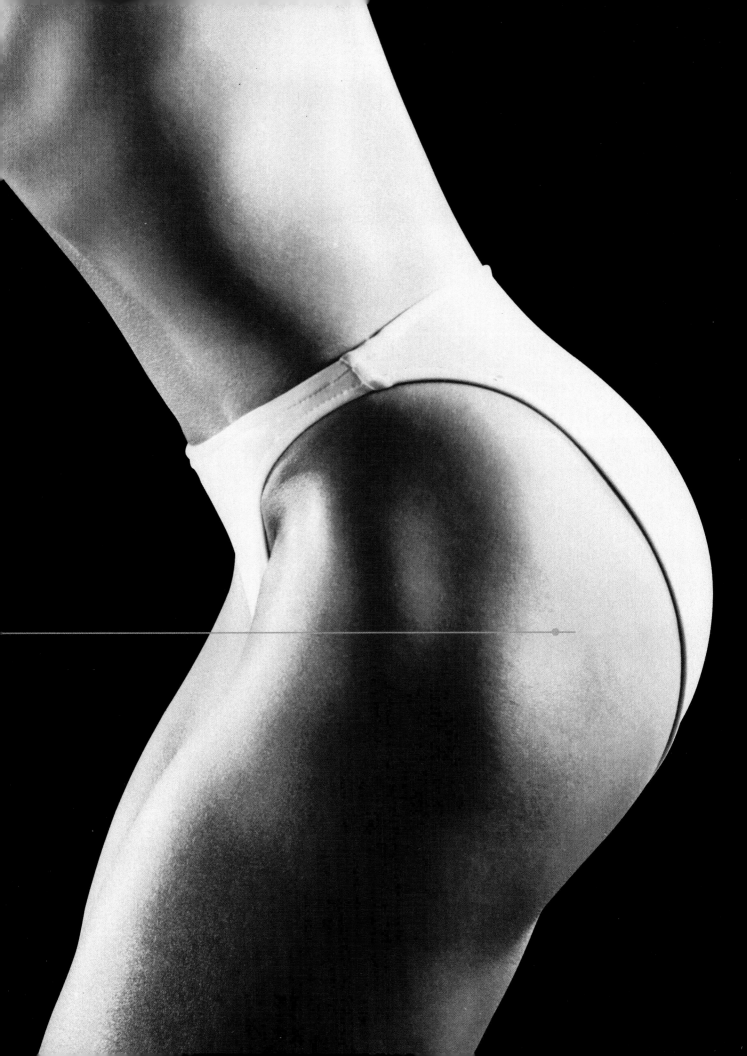

BUTTOCKS A firm, tight butt not only turns heads but is a sure sign of a well-conditioned individual. The strong muscles of the buttocks are our power center, enabling us to sprint, jump, and perform other dynamic moves. Conditioned buttocks also help prevent knee and back injuries. | With regard to training, there are two distinct groups: Those of us who want to build up our buttocks, and those of us who desperately want to decrease the size of our backsides. To build more rounded, shapely buttocks you must concentrate on extension and rotation exercises that work the buttocks at the deepest layers. Squatting exercises should be performed with a full range of motion, lowering until the upper legs go parallel with the floor. | Have you ever noticed that the buttocks of track athletes are not only fat-free but highly developed? It's no accident; it's the result of sprinting and jumping drills. To add more muscularity to your gluteals, first perform the compound exercises in this chapter, then practice the additional jumping and lunging drills. When climbing stairs, exaggerate the height of your stride and try climbing two steps at a time with your hands behind your head. | Refining the buttocks to decrease size requires high-frequency, low-intensity exercise. This means you need to work your buttocks every training day. First perform my compound exercises, increasing the repetitions as you progress. Then perform the low intensity moves provided in this chapter. Aerobic activities are ideal because they combine long duration with light intensity and emphasis on the lower body. In a step class, always step with your weight on your heel first, then squeeze your buttocks as you raise up. | If you use a stairclimber, get added benefit by standing up straight, not leaning forward. Shorten your stride so you can step at a brisk pace and you'll feel the intensity not only in your buttocks, but also in your legs.

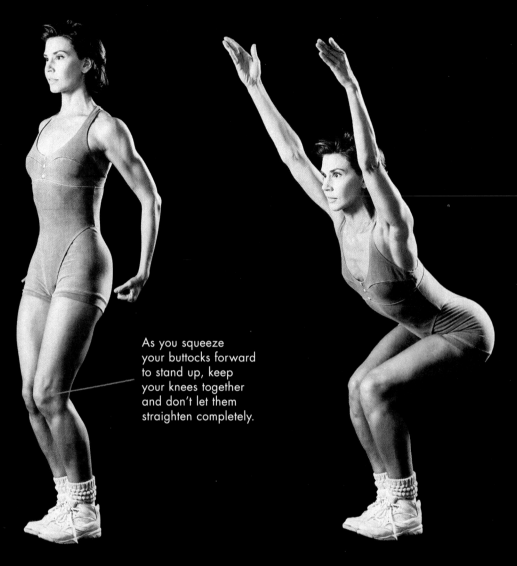

As you squeeze your buttocks forward to stand up, keep your knees together and don't let them straighten completely.

feet together
half-up squat   *(gluteals, quadriceps, hamstrings)*

a Stand with your feet, knees, and ankles together. Bend your arms slightly, allowing your hands to start near your hips. Bend your knees slightly, bringing your buttocks forward over your heels.

b Bend your knees even more until your buttocks are sitting behind your heels. Extend your arms overhead without dropping your chest. Squeeze your buttocks forward over your heels and raise up slightly. Return to the start and repeat for 16 repetitions.

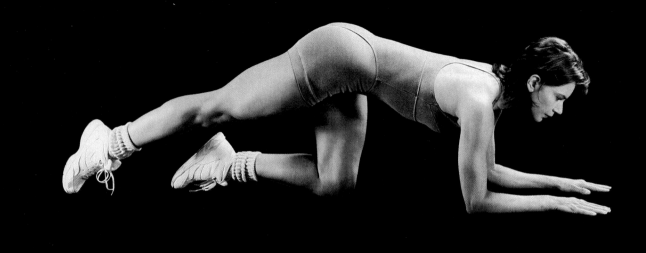

Do not let your hips rotate as you lift the leg — your hips should remain square to the floor, rotating the thigh at the hip.

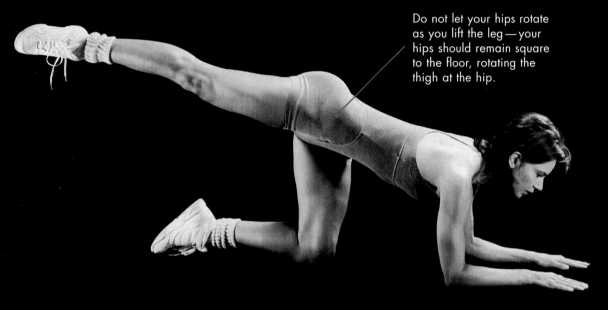

leg rotation *(gluteus maximus, gluteus minimus, piriformis)*

a Kneel down on your elbows and left knee with your right leg extended behind you. Your toes should be touching the floor.

b Lift your straight leg up to hip level and simultaneously rotate your thigh outward. Hold this position for two seconds before lowering down to a parallel position. Perform 16 repetitions and repeat using the other leg.

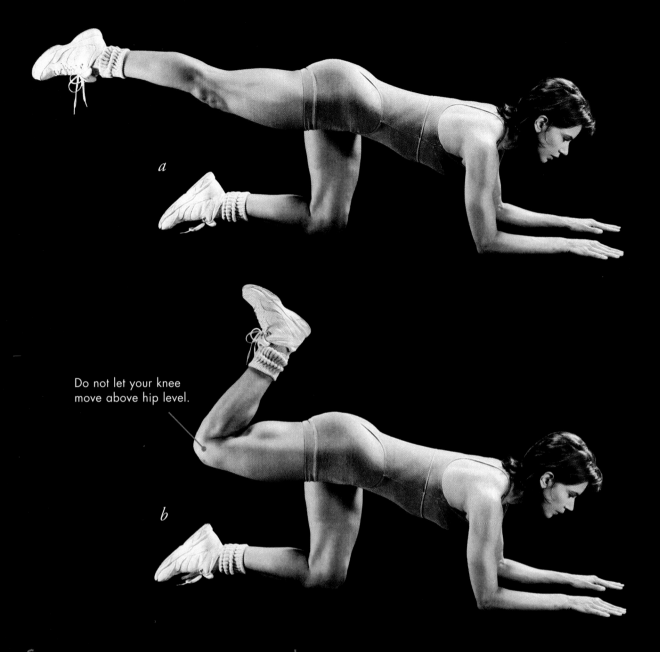

a

Do not let your knee
move above hip level.

b

four-part curl *(gluteals, hamstrings, quadriceps)*

ⓐ Kneel down on your elbows and left knee, with your left thigh perpendicular to the floor. Straighten your right leg and hold it up at hip level to the floor. Look straight down and point your toes.

ⓑ Flex your foot and bend your right knee, squeezing the hamstring muscle to bring the heel toward the buttocks. Keep your knee stationary.

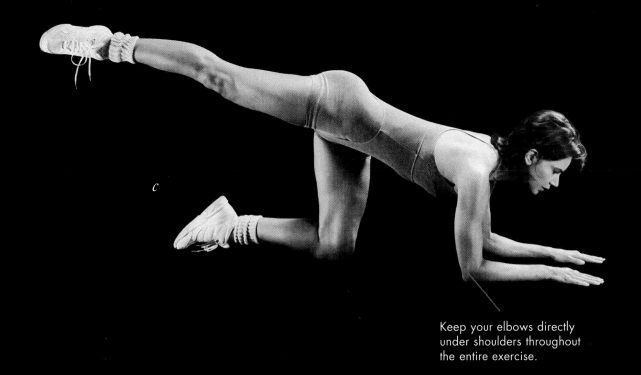

c

Keep your elbows directly under shoulders throughout the entire exercise.

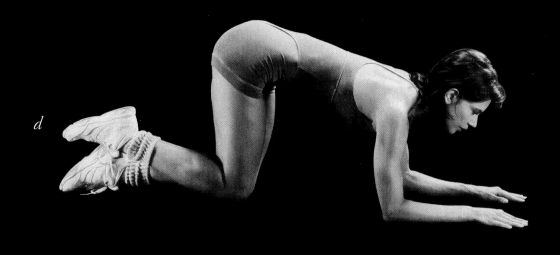

d

ⓒ Extend your leg out again, straight behind you.

ⓓ Bring your right knee down to meet your left knee, keeping your torso straight and your abdominals pulled in to support your back. Pause for a two count in each of the four positions. Repeat this sequence 12 times for each leg.

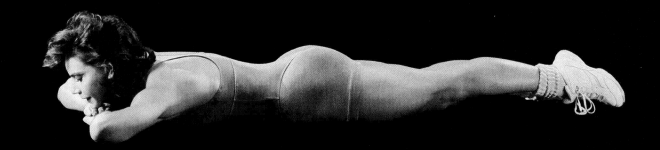

Keep your lifting leg
absolutely straight and in a
parallel position. This works
the area where the buttocks
connect to the hamstrings.

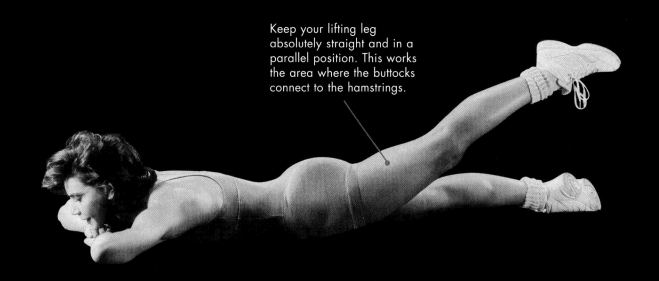

rear leg lifts   *(gluteals – low intensity)*

a   Lie face down with your legs straight
back and your hands folded in front of
you, resting your chin in your hands.

b   While keeping your torso in contact
with the floor, lift your left leg as high as
possible without allowing your hips or
shoulders to twist. Pause for two seconds
and then return to the start. Perform 16
repetitions, working to 24 reps, then
repeat with the other leg.

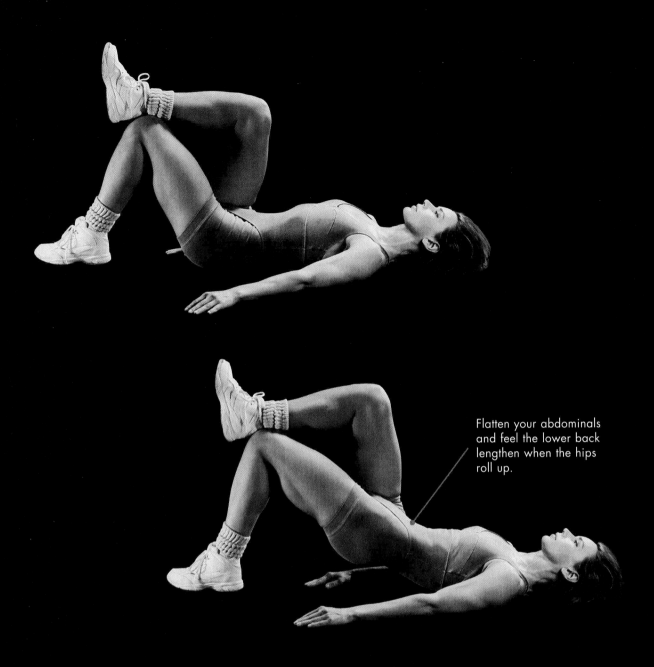

Flatten your abdominals and feel the lower back lengthen when the hips roll up.

butt tucks *(gluteals — low intensity)*

a Lie on your back, place your hands at your sides, and bend your left knee, foot flat on the floor. Place your right ankle on the left knee — this increases the weight over the bottom leg.

b Press your back against the floor and squeeze the buttocks to roll your hips off the floor. Hold the top of each contraction for two seconds. Don't lift your head. Perform 24 to 36 reps and repeat for the other side.

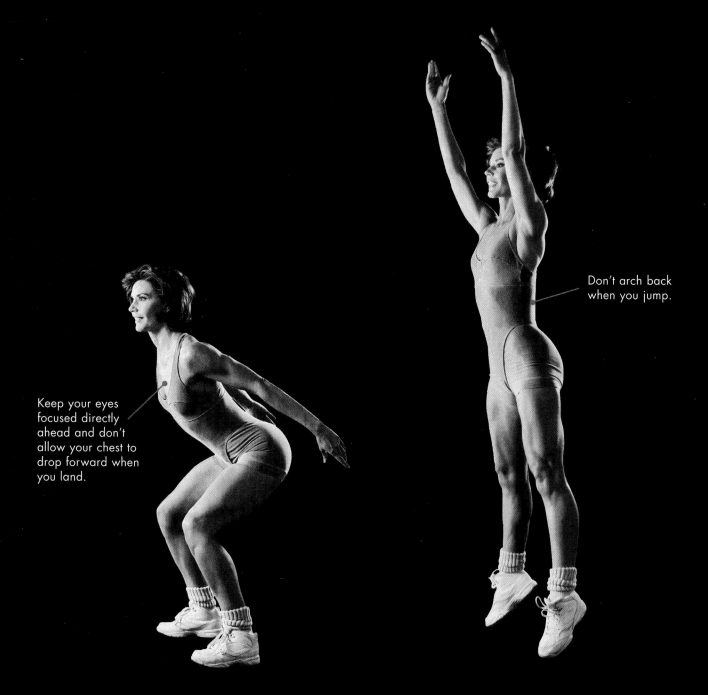

Don't arch back
when you jump.

Keep your eyes
focused directly
ahead and don't
allow your chest to
drop forward when
you land.

butt builder   *(gluteals, thighs, calves—high intensity)*

a Stand with your legs shoulder-width apart. Bend your knees until your hips are behind your heels. Sit back into the buttocks and extend your arms back.

b Jump as high as possible while swinging your arms up; land softly by absorbing the impact with the ball of your foot, then the heel. (This technique minimizes the stress on your knees.) Pause for two seconds at the bottom before repeating. Perform ten repetitions.

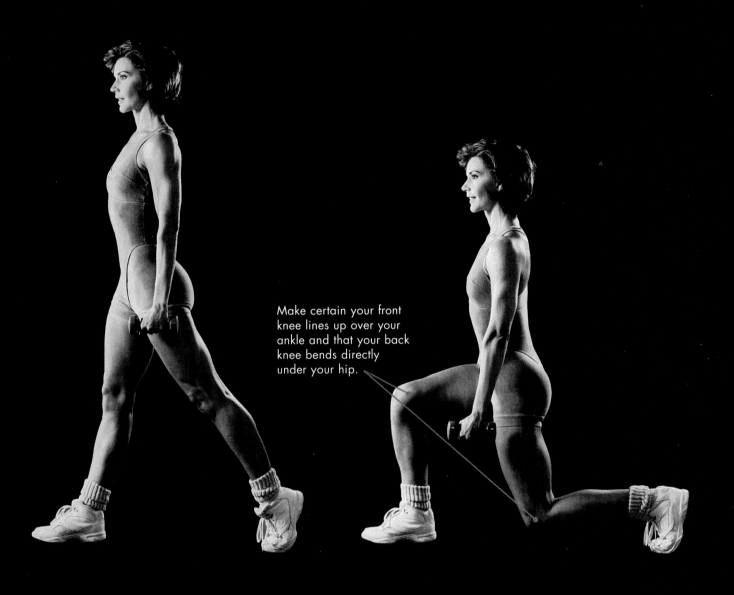

Make certain your front knee lines up over your ankle and that your back knee bends directly under your hip.

scissor lunges *(gluteals, thighs – high intensity)*

a Hold three-to-five-pound hand weights with one leg forward and the other leg back about three feet (less if you are shorter and more if you are taller). Balance on the ball of the rear foot.

b Bend your knees until your rear knee almost touches the floor. Keeping your back straight up. To come out of the lunge, push down against the front leg heel and squeeze your buttocks tight. Perform 16 repetitions and then repeat for the other side.

DEFINED abdominals

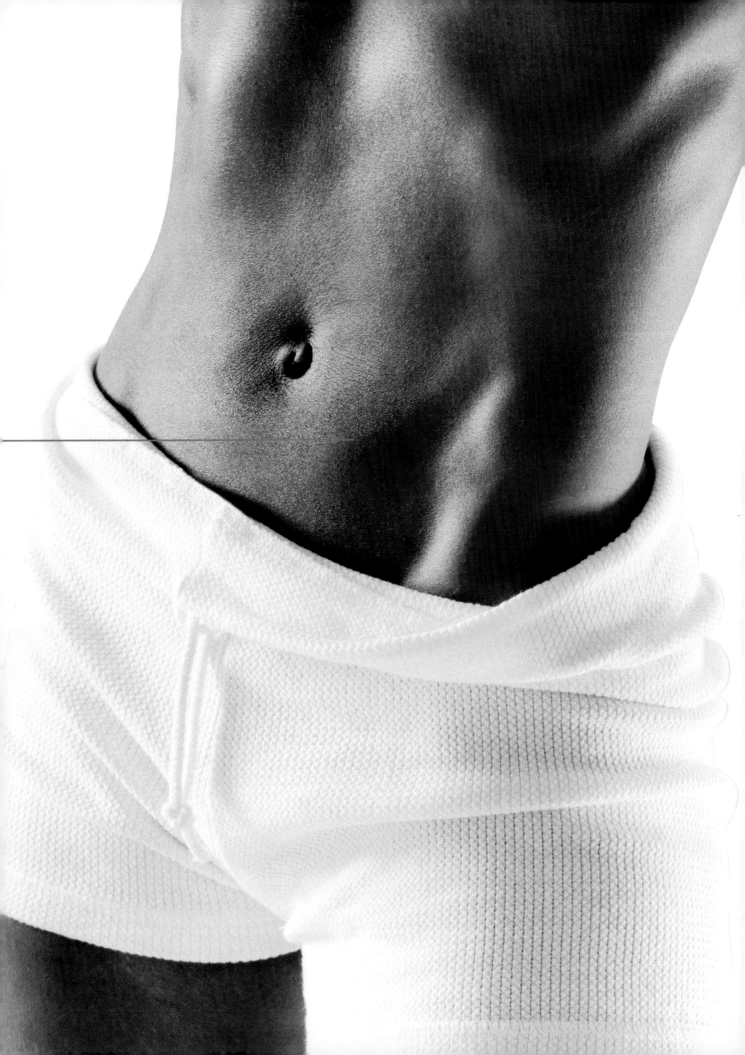

ABDOMINALS A trim midsection with visible abdominal muscles is the icing on the cake for most health and fitness enthusiasts. They not only look good, but achieving definition in the front of the torso means you have both good abdominal development and a very low percentage of body fat. | Whether you see them or not, we all have abdominals — without these stabilizing muscles of the torso we would not be able to sit up. The problem is that most people's enviable abs are covered with a layer of flab. Therefore, your abdominal routine must be accompanied by low-fat, sensible eating habits in order to achieve that lean, chiseled look. | Abdominal exercise is unique. Unlike exercising your arms and legs, which require expansive movements, the actual movements for the abs are very small and extremely precise. | When training your abdominals it is especially important that you "feel" each repetition and concentrate on the muscles contracting. One of the most important goals of abdominal training is to create a balanced working relationship between all areas of the abs. This includes attention to the lower and upper regions of the rectus abdominis, the obliques, and the transversus abdominis. | Contrary to some beliefs, the rectus abdominis is not made of two different muscles. It is one long sheath comprised of various muscle fibers. Specific exercises will focus on the upper or lower fibers, allowing you to target particular regions. The obliques are responsible for rotating the spine. The transversus abdominis is the muscle you use to "pull your stomach in." Together these muscles bend and twist the spine and flatten the abdomen. | To prepare for abdominal training begin with a stretching movement to loosen the lower back. This helps you isolate the abdominal muscles better and minimizes back tension, which can limit your full range of motion. The pelvic tilt

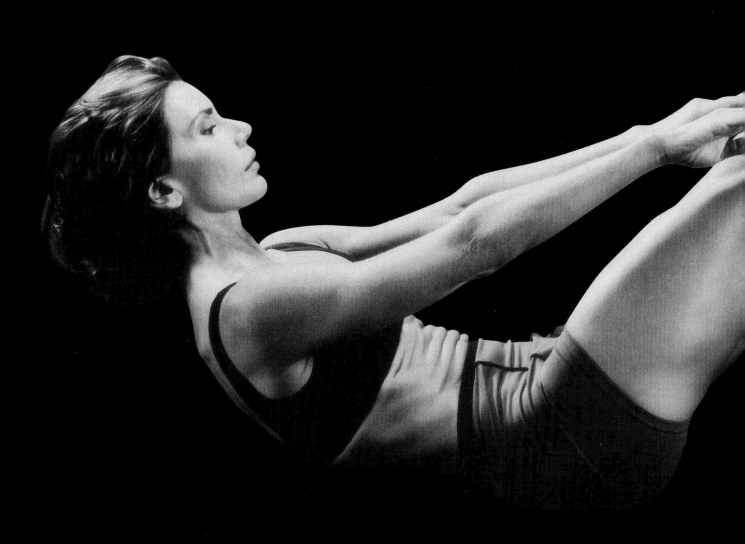

in the previous buttocks chapter is a good way to stretch your back. | In all sit-up movements, relax your pelvis and press your lower back to the floor. Rather than pushing outward toward the abdominal wall, contract the abdominals inward toward your spine. Think of creating a C-shape to your torso. Use your abs to actually suspend your shoulders and pelvis in a slight upward arc. Throughout this abdominal routine, practice slow, steady, and controlled breathing with each repetition. Inhale as you prepare for the movement, exhale as you perform the movement — at the peak of the contraction make sure you have fully exhaled. Follow these guidelines and you'll be on your way to awesome abs.

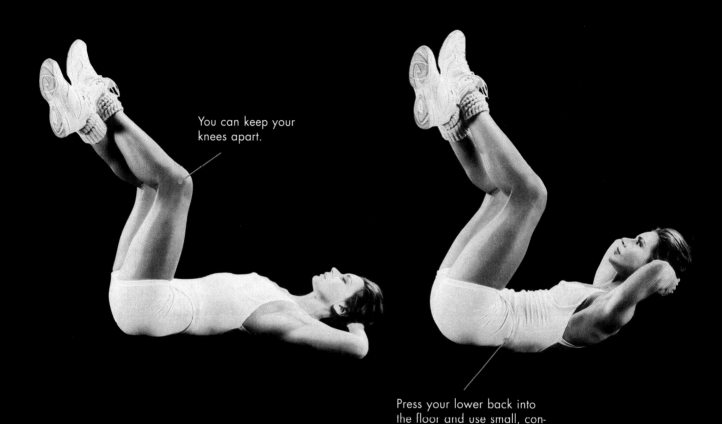

You can keep your knees apart.

Press your lower back into the floor and use small, controlled movements to raise your hips and shoulders.

double crunch *(rectus abdominis, transversus, obliques)*

(a) Lie on your back with legs up, ankles crossed and your knees bent. Place your hands behind your head and point your elbows out.

(b) Squeeze your abdominals, pressing your lower back into the floor. Curl your shoulders off the ground and simultaneously roll your hips toward your chest. Pause at the top of the curl, then slowly unroll to the starting position, resting your head on the floor after each repetition.

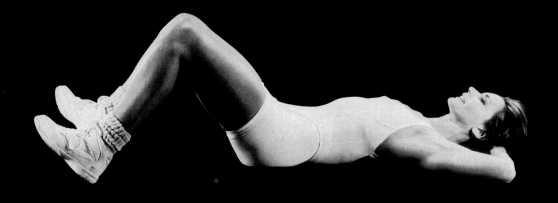

Do not swing your elbows forward and yank on your head. This places harmful stress on the neck.

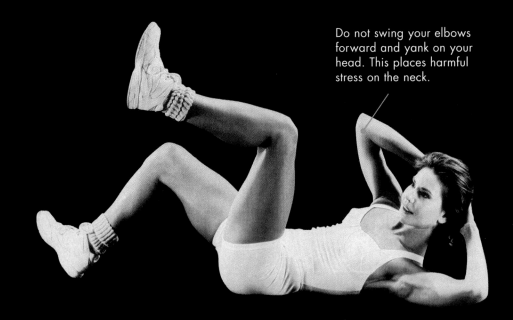

alternate
elbow-to-knee *(obliques, transversus, rectus abdominis)*

(a) Lie on your back with your hands behind your head and elbows pointed out. Bend your knees and rest on your heels.

(b) Squeeze the sides of your abdominals while lifting your left knee. Cross your right shoulder towards the lifted knee. The right shoulder should be lifted off the floor while you hips remain flat. Pause for two seconds, return to the start and repeat for the other side. Alternate legs until you have performed 12 repetitions on each side.

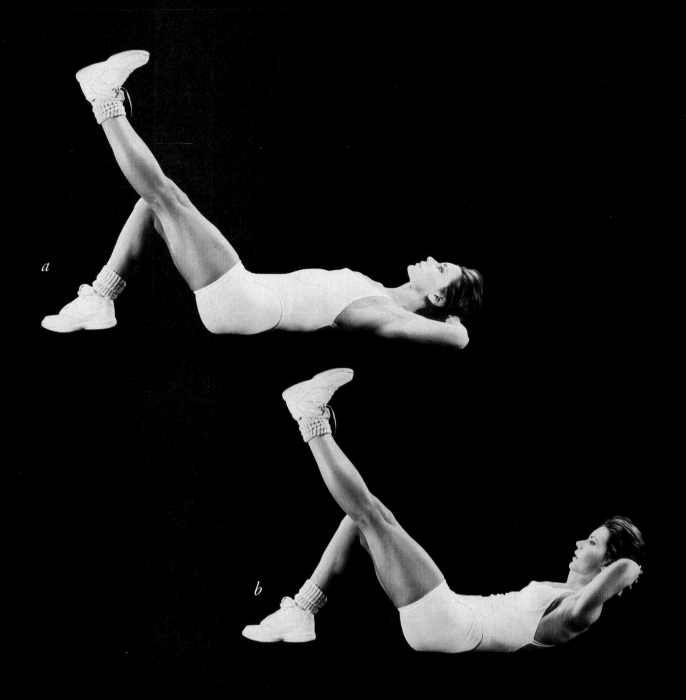

curl and reach *(rectus abdominis, transversus abdominis)*

a Lie on your back. Bending your right knee, extend your left leg to a 45-degree angle with a flexed foot. Place your hands behind your head, pressing your back against the floor.

b Holding the leg stationary, curl your torso so that your shoulders come off the floor.

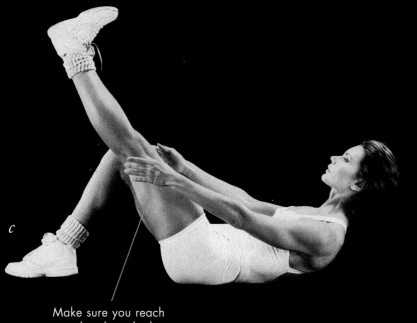

c

Make sure you reach
your hands to the knee
without letting that leg
move up and away
from the other leg.

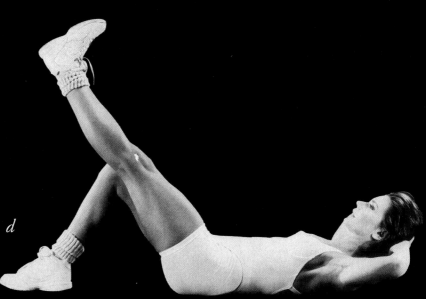

d

(c) Increase the curl as you reach your hands toward your knees.

(d) Place your hands behind your head and slowly roll down to release.

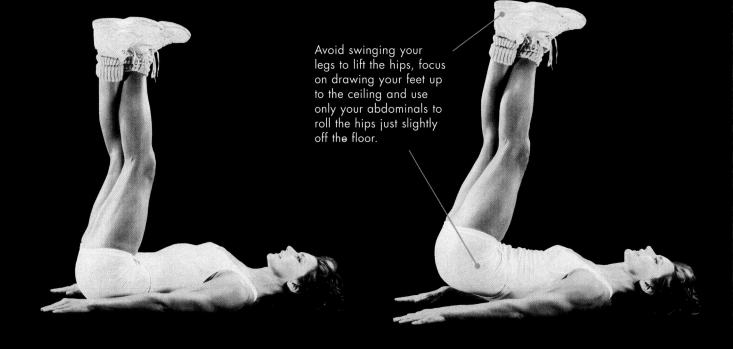

Avoid swinging your legs to lift the hips, focus on drawing your feet up to the ceiling and use only your abdominals to roll the hips just slightly off the floor.

reverse curls *(rectus abdominis)*

a Lie face up and place both hands at your sides, head resting on the floor. Cross your ankles and hold your legs in the air, knees slightly bent. Before you begin, press your abdominals toward the floor.

b Without lifting your head, raise your hips slightly off the floor until your buttocks and tailbone clear. Pause at the top and then slowly return to the start. Perform 12 repetitions.

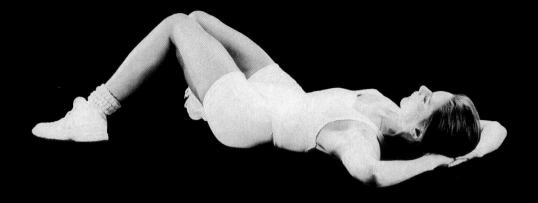

Visualize leading with your
shoulder and extending
your hand past your leg to
intensify the contraction.

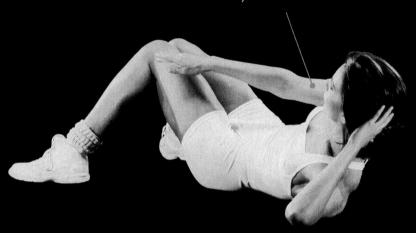

cross crunch *(obliques)*

a   Lie face up and place both hands behind your head. Bend and bring your knees together, feet apart and flat on the floor.

b   Begin by curling the right shoulder up and across until your shoulder blade lifts off the floor. Reach your right hand to the left knee, pause, and then return to the start position, placing your hands behind your head and resting your head on the floor each time. Complete 16 repetitions and repeat on the other side.

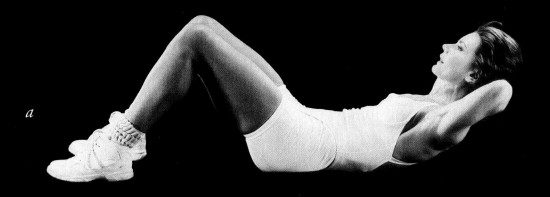

a

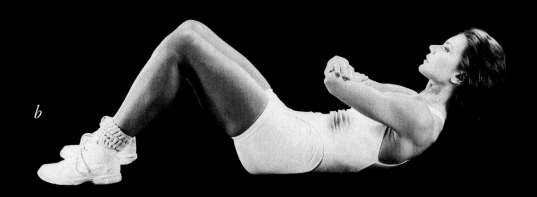

b

10-5-5-10 series *(rectus abdominis, transversus abdominis)*

(*a*) Lie face up, bend your knees, and place your hands behind your head but do not clasp them. Flare your elbows out. Press your abdominals toward the floor and curl your torso up and forward. Pause for two seconds and then return to the start. Perform ten repetitions.

(*b*) Perform a second set with your hands across your elbows. Curl your torso up and forward, squeezing your abdominals and leading with your elbows and chest. Pause for two seconds before returning to the start. Perform five repetitions.

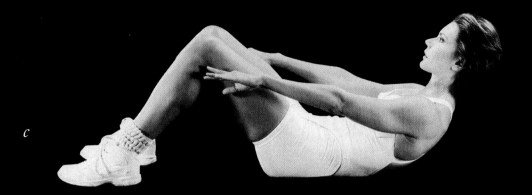

c

Relax your pelvis so your back is on the floor. Exhale at the peak of each curl.

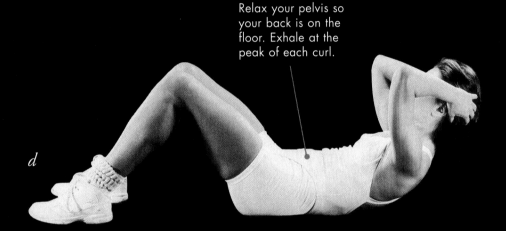

d

c The third set is with your hands reaching front. Keep your chin stationary, and if your neck gets tired place one hand behind your head. Perform five repetitions.

d Do the last 10 reps with fingertips on the side of the head, elbows facing front. Curl your torso forward and press your abdominals down.

SENSUOUS back

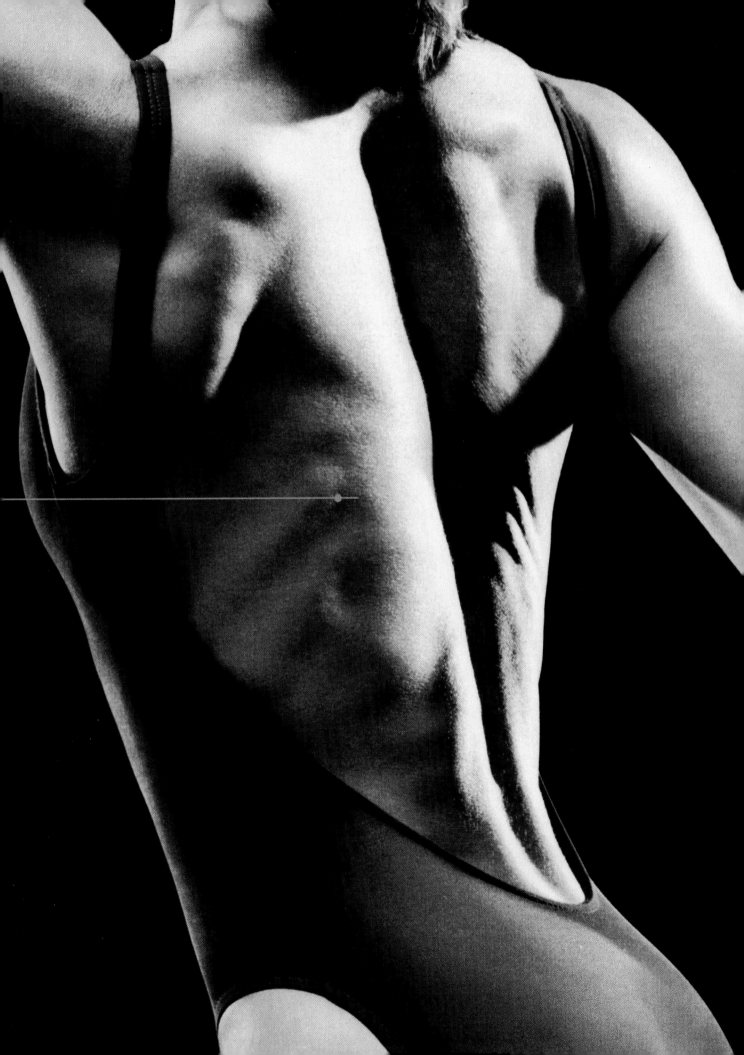

BACK The backs of ballerinas and swimmers are often artfully sculpted, symmetrical, and agile. In addition to the beauty of a well-developed back, conditioning this dramatic muscle group is essential to maintaining an attractive posture. | Test your posture. If your shoulders are rounded and posture hunched forward, the space between your shoulder blades may be six to eight inches apart. If your posture is good and your upper back muscles properly balanced with your chest and shoulders, this space should be only four to six inches. | Poor posture when sitting, standing, and walking tends to weaken the supportive structure of the back. The exercise routine I've created requires you to spend nearly as much time on your back muscles as you do on your abdominals and the muscles of the front of your body in order to correct potential imbalances. | As opposed to the "mirror muscles" in the chest and shoulders, the back is made up of many layers of small muscles that work together to bend, twist, and lift. | The upper back is powerful, providing a base of strength for your arms and shoulders. The lower back is equally important to stabilize and protect the base of the spinal column. The lower back is often a place where people feel stress and hold nervous tension. This is also an area that fatigues easily. By performing these exercises you will build muscular strength, endurance, and balance in your entire back, improve your posture, and help to prevent potential back problems and associate pain. With careful and consistent training, a defined, athletic-looking back is attainable at any age in a short amount of time

As you round your back, roll your shoulders forward and pull your abdominals up and in to increase the stretch.

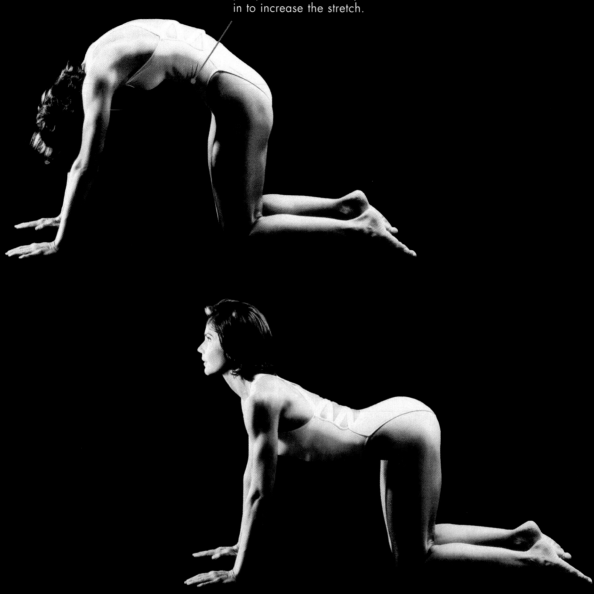

cat move *(entire back)*

ⓐ Support yourself on your hands and knees. Place your hands about shoulder-width apart and directly underneath your shoulders. Place your knees directly under your hips with your thighs perpendicular to the floor. Start by tucking your chin into your chest and rounding your entire back. Exhale and hold for a four count.

ⓑ Inhale and arch your back, lifting your chin gently and holding for a four count while exhaling. Make sure you don't sit back toward your feet. Continue bowing and arching your back in this manner for ten repetitions.

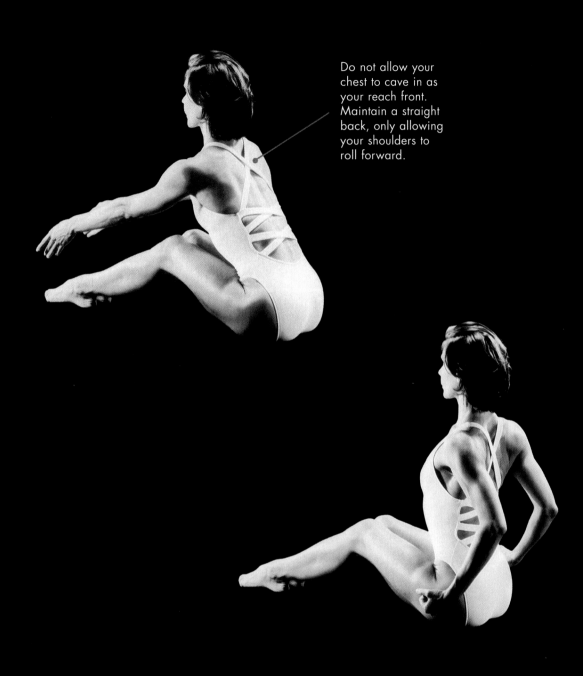

Do not allow your chest to cave in as your reach front. Maintain a straight back, only allowing your shoulders to roll forward.

seated rows *(entire back)*

(a) Sit upright with your legs extended in front of you, knees slightly bent. Lean forward from the hips and reach your hands to your feet. Keep your chest lifted and your abdominals pulled in.

(b) Tensing your back, wrap your arms and shoulders back. Lift your chest and squeeze your shoulder blades together. Your palms should be facing up and your elbows should extend about six to eight inches behind your back. Hold this position for two seconds before returning to the start. Perform 12 repetitions and work up to 16.

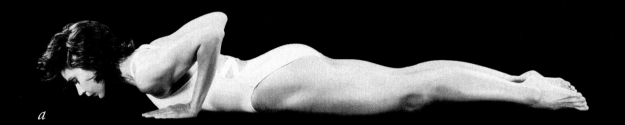

a

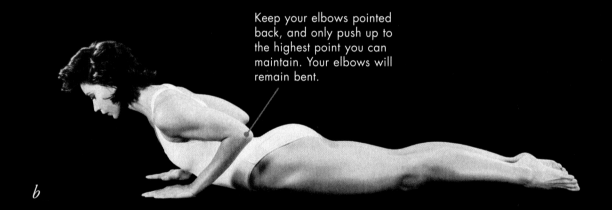

Keep your elbows pointed
back, and only push up to
the highest point you can
maintain. Your elbows will
remain bent.

b

push and holds *(entire back)*

(a) Lie face down and place your hands at the sides of your chest as if you were going to perform a push-up.

(b) Keep your hips in full contact with the floor and use your arms to push your chest a few inches off the floor. Keep you head in line with your spine by looking down.

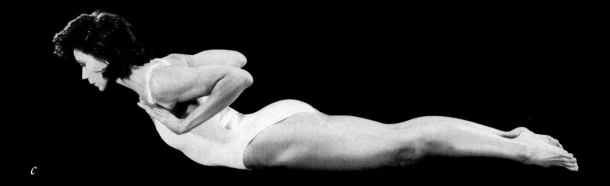

c

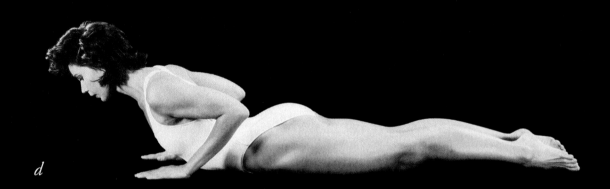

d

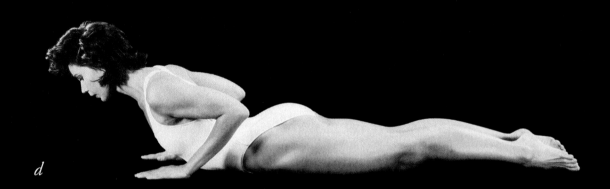

c   Tense your back muscles to hold your chest up so you can lift your hands several inches off the floor without dropping your chest.

d   Return your hands to the start position and lower your chest to the floor. Perform for eight reps and eventually progress to 12 reps.

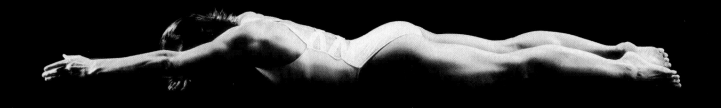

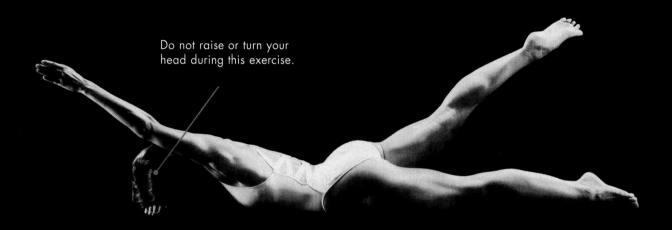

Do not raise or turn your
head during this exercise.

alternate
leg-arm extensions *(entire back)*

(a) Lie face down, resting your forehead on your right hand. Extend your left arm out with the thumb facing up.

(b) Lift your left hand and right leg off the floor. Hold for two seconds before lowering to the floor. Perform eight repetitions and repeat for the other side. Complete two sets on each side.

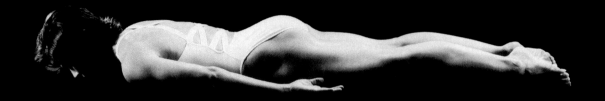

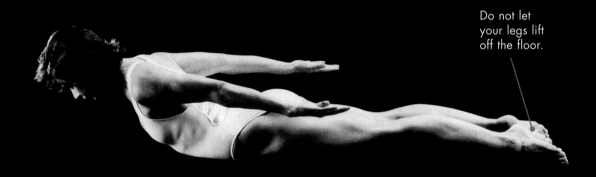

Do not let your legs lift off the floor.

swan squeeze *(entire back)*

a Lie face down with your hands at your sides, palms up.

b Lift your chest off the floor, keeping your chin tucked in so that you're looking down. Lift your chest and hands as high as possible and squeeze your shoulder blades together. Hold for four seconds and then slowly lower down to the start. Perform 10 repetitions.

SUPPLE stretch

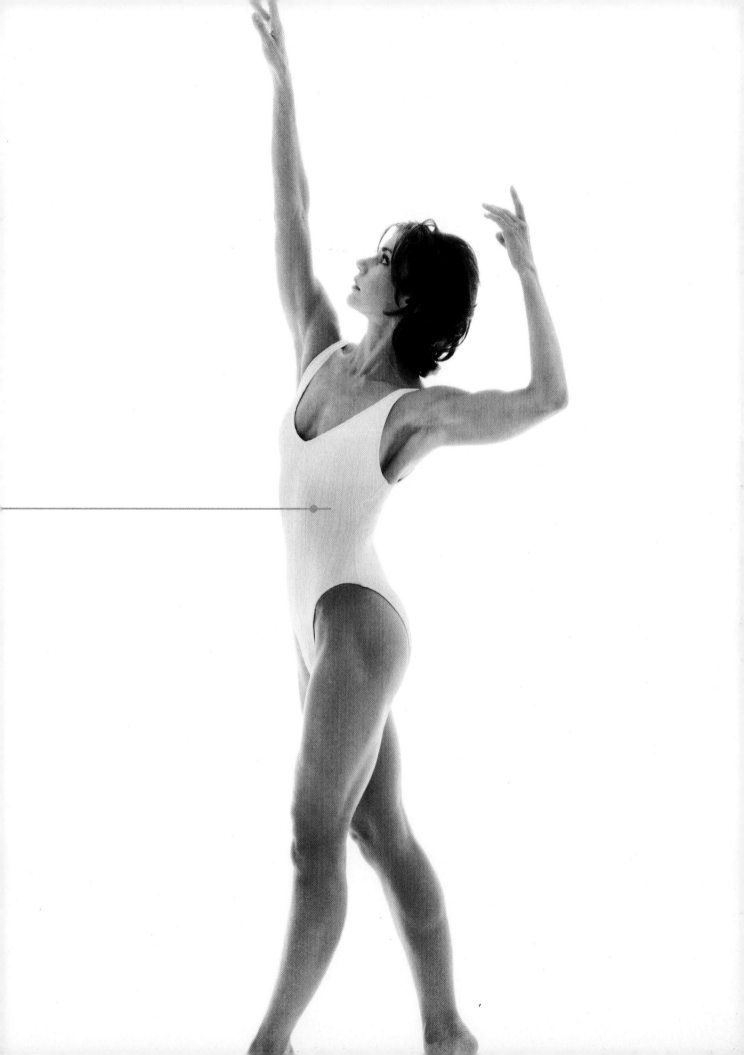

A yoga instructor once described stretching to me as "letting your body speak." As you stretch, open up these communication lines between your body and mind. Concentrate on "feeling" the muscles — not just the large ones you can see moving, but the smaller ones as well. Always stretch slowly; it encourages a calm, peaceful, and almost meditative state. I like to stretch with soft music after a workout to let not only my muscles relax but my mind as well.

THE THREE R's OF STRETCHING

RELAXATION Before beginning your stretches, take a few moments to relax. Adopt a comfortable position. You shouldn't feel stiff or awkward. Find your natural level of flexibility with each stretch.

RESPIRATION Always breathe deeply and evenly. Exhale slowly through your nose and feel your body relax.

RELEASE Relaxation and respiration create a physical and an emotional release. You can enhance this feeling by using visualization techniques. As you hold the stretch, imagine your muscles like warm butter, melting and softening. Float with the feeling as your muscles release and elongate. At the conclusion, enjoy the sensation and look of your muscles in their more supple, vital, and energized state.

STRETCHING TIPS

- Warm up for at least five minutes before stretching, or stretch at the end of your workout routine. Warm, loose muscles are more pliable than cold, tight muscles.

- Always stretch in a warm, comfortable environment. Avoid drafty areas and cold rooms.

- Stretch on carpet or use a towel mat for padding.

- Don't wear clothing, shoes, or belts that restrict your range of motion.

- Never force your body to extremes.

- Ease into your maximum comfortable stretch position then hold it for at least 30 seconds.

- You should feel a tightness in the muscle, but not in the joint. If you feel stress in the joint, alleviate it by modifying your position.

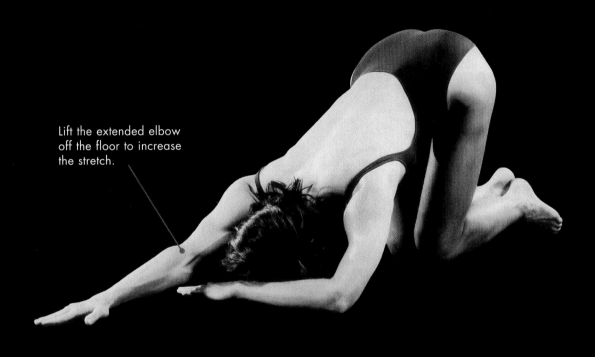

Lift the extended elbow
off the floor to increase
the stretch.

shoulder stretch

_a_ Begin from an "all fours" position with your knees together. Extend one arm and bend
the other arm. Rest your forehead on the floor. Shift your hips back toward your feet
until you feel a stretch in your shoulder and back. Hold this position for 15 seconds.
Repeat with the other arm extended.

Feel your arms reaching away from your feet, but don't let your hips raise off the floor.

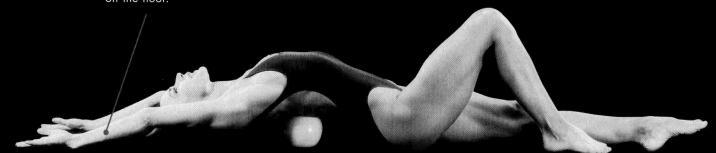

spine lengthener

a) Lie face up, place a ball under your shoulder blades, extend both arms out. Bend your right knee with the foot flat on the floor. Extend your left leg out and point your foot. Lengthen your body as much as possible while arching your back away from the floor; breathe, and relax. Hold this position for 15 seconds. Repeat by bending the left knee and holding for 15 seconds.

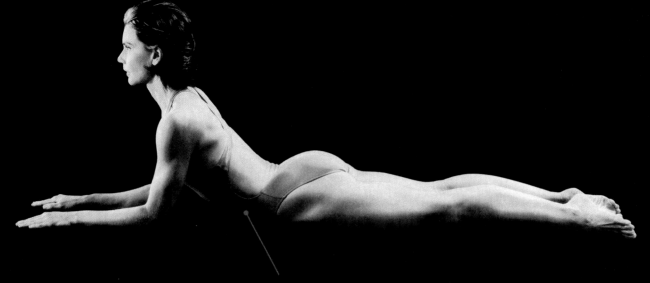

For an extra stretch you can lift your left elbow up slightly to stretch the left side abdominals. Hold for 15 seconds, then repeat for the other side.

abdominal stretch

a   Lie face down with your legs straight behind you. Prop yourself up so that your elbows are slightly forward of your shoulders.

b   Keep your hips in full contact with the floor. Stretch the front of your torso and feel your rib cage lengthening from your hip bones. Relax, breathe, and hold this position for 30 seconds.

Do not let your knees
spread apart — they
should remain in line
with your hips.

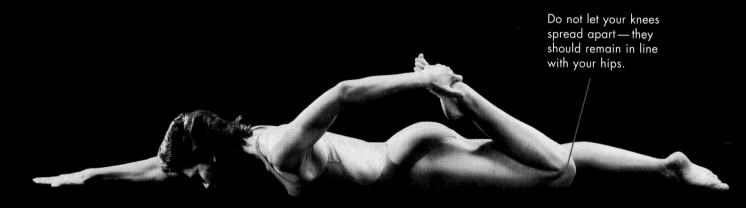

quad stretch

a   Lie face down with your right leg out straight behind you. Bend your left knee and grasp
the top of your foot with your left hand. Keeping your hips in contact with the floor,
bring your heel to your buttocks. Tuck your buttocks to emphasize the stretch in the front
of the thigh. Hold for 30 seconds, and then slowly return to the start before stretching
the other leg.

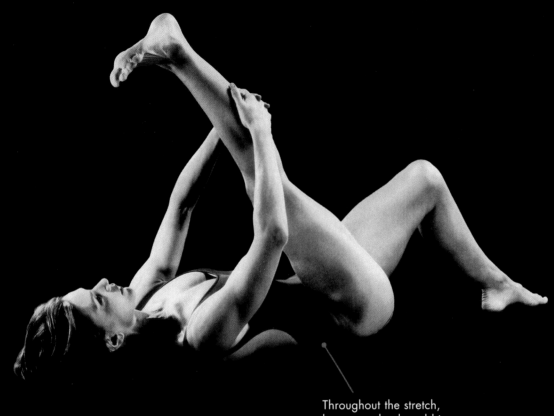

Throughout the stretch,
keep your back and hips
in contact with the floor.

hamstring stretch

a Lie face up with your left leg bent, foot flat on the floor. Holding your calf, bring your right leg as far forward as possible toward your head without bending your knee. When you've attained the maximum stretch in the back of your right thigh, breathe and hold for 30 seconds, slowly lower the leg to the floor and repeat with the other leg.

Do not round or twist your upper back — your back should be straight with your chest lifted, rotate your torso from the hips.

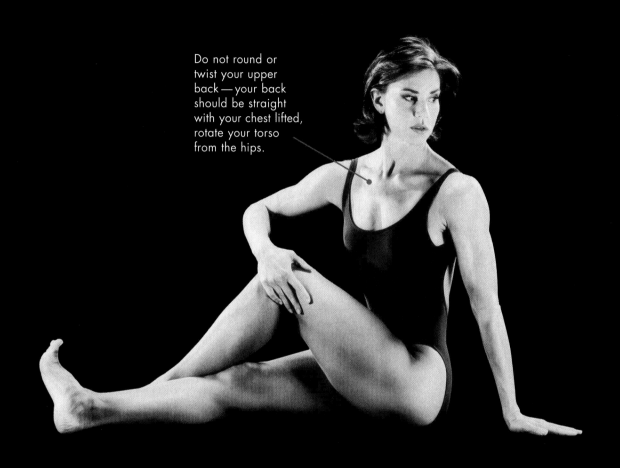

low back stretch

a   Sit upright with your back straight and right leg extended in front of you. Bend and cross your left leg over your right. Now rotate your torso to the left and and look over your left shoulder. Hold for 30 seconds and then repeat for the other side. You should feel a good stretch in your lower back.

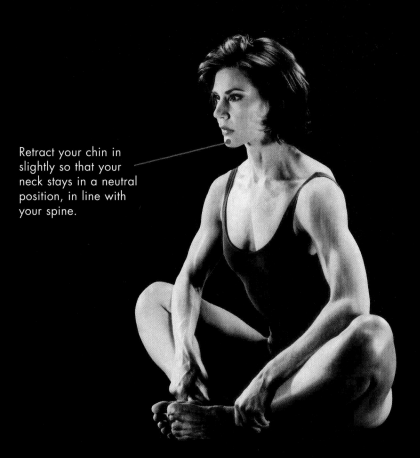

Retract your chin in slightly so that your neck stays in a neutral position, in line with your spine.

butterfly

a Sit on the floor, grasp your ankles, and press the soles of your feet together. Rest your elbows against the inside of your thighs and lean forward from the hips. Keep your back straight and chest lifted to feel the inner thigh stretch. Enhance the stretch by pressing your knees down as far as comfortable, hold for 30 seconds, and then relax.

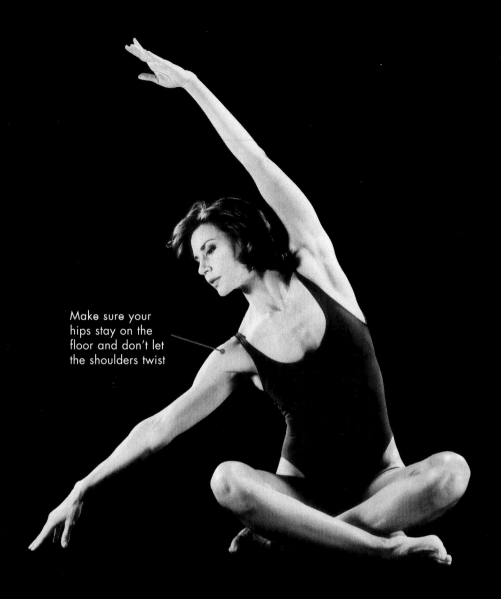

Make sure your hips stay on the floor and don't let the shoulders twist

dancer's stretch

(a) Sit on the floor and cross your legs so that your left leg is in front. Reach your left hand to the side, in line with your hips, and then extend your right arm overhead. Lean to your left. Turn your chin to the left and glance down. You should feel a continuous stretch from your right hip to your right hand. Hold a comfortable stretch for 30 seconds, return to center, then change legs and repeat for the other side.

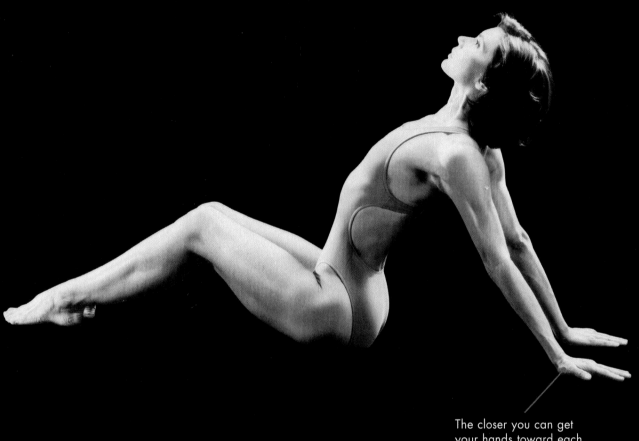

The closer you can get your hands toward each other, the more you will feel the stretch in your chest and shoulders.

dolphin stretch

(*a*) Sit on the floor. Bend your knees with your feet flat on the floor in front of you. Walk your hands behind you with your fingers pointed away from your body. Lift your rib cage up, press your chest forward and wrap your shoulders back. Look up slightly as you do this. You should feel the stretch in your chest, shoulders, and arms. Hold for 30 seconds.

SAFETY matters

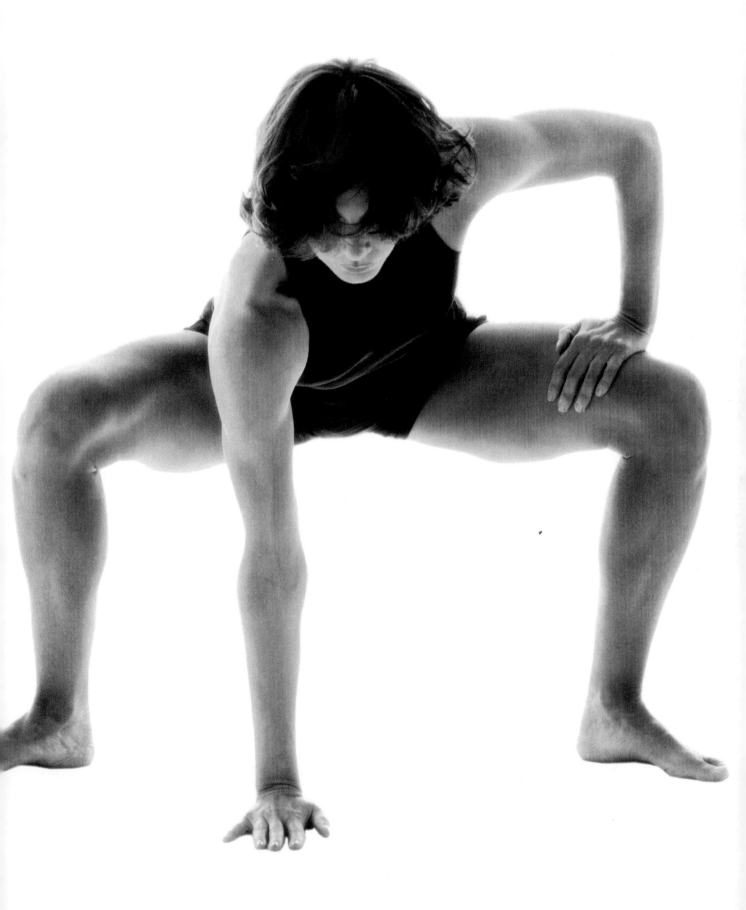

BEING ON A SOUND FITNESS PROGRAM PUTS YOU ON THE CUTTING EDGE OF HEALTH.

Certainly the exterior changes—strong muscles and a lean body—are important. The internal feelings of accomplishment and self-confidence are equally important. But the fact that exercise improves our general health may be the best reason of all to do it.

Along with improving cardiovascular fitness for a healthier heart, exercise lowers cholesterol in the blood to further reduce the risk of developing heart disease. It also helps prevent adult-onset diabetes, hypertension, and certain cancers. Of particular importance to women, exercise slows the loss of bone mass (osteoporosis) associated with aging.

A well-conditioned body helps internal organs function more efficiently. By stretching and strengthening the muscles of the torso you can improve your digestion and protect your spine for better neurological function. The

improved circulation and blood flow gives you more energy, increases your stamina, and helps you wake up faster and go to sleep easier. A proper exercise program not only strengthens the body's stabilizing muscles for better posture, but it also helps you avoid and correct some of the common problems that arise from a sedentary lifestyle, including back pain. More than $50 billion a year is spent on medical care for the treatment of back pain. The incidence of back injury is even higher in people who perform sports related activities that involve throwing, jumping, and running. Some theorists blame the high incidence of back pain on the fact that we stand erect, claiming that our upright stance is inferior to the posture of other mammals, such as a dog. This is simply not true. Four-legged animals have an inherent structural weakness in the middle of the spine, whereas our columnlike structure is better suited for weight bearing. What is true is that one of the primary factors to blame for the epidemic of back pain is poor posture.

Ideal posture is a healthy balance between the muscular and skeletal systems. Take this simple test: Stand with your back, buttocks, heels, shoulders, and head against the wall, and try to slide your hand through your back at belt-line level. If you have a normal arch, the thickest part of your hand will just fill the gap between the wall and your back. If your hand slides right through you have too much curvature and need to strengthen your abdominals and stretch your back muscles. If your fingers barely fit in the gap, you have too little curvature and need to focus on back extension exercises.

One factor affecting posture is your height. If you're short, you tend to adjust to your environment by looking up. This posture increases the arch in your back. Wearing high-heeled shoes also forces the body to exaggerate this arch, along with causing unnatural bending in the hips, knees, and neck.

If you're tall, you tend to adjust to your environment by looking down. This posture causes you to round your shoulders, flatten your back, and thrust your pelvis forward. The center of gravity changes in this position, causing a pot

belly appearance in the lower abdomen. This posture may eventually contribute to a hump in the upper back, and if left untreated can degenerate to the point where it cannot be corrected. If caught early and treated with the back exercises presented in this program, this condition can often be corrected.

The best course of action to improve your posture and avoid related problems is to develop a strong, stable back. Keep in mind, however, that a strong back requires strong abdominals, and here's why: The abdominals provide the muscular link between the upper body and the lower body. They need to be strong enough to support the spine through the constant bending, lifting, pulling, pushing, and twisting motions of everyday life. If they are weak and fatigue easily, they are not able to hold the pelvis in correct alignment, which then creates postural problems and related back pain.

Think of your torso as the trunk of a tree that acts as the foundation for all the branches. A torso that has strong, balanced abdominal and back muscles becomes the solid base of support for our limbs and allows them to move freely without injury to the back.

To get the most out of your torso-training exercises while keeping them safe, here's what to remember:

1 Practice good posture when you're standing, sitting, and walking. Hold your head high — think of raising your head up into a crown. Lift your chest and pull your abdominals in, keeping your hips in a neutral position.

2 If you need to lift a heavy object from the floor, squat down and straddle the load. Keep the chest lifted, knees bent, and hips centered. Lift the object using the strength of your arms, legs, and buttocks — think of pushing your legs down through the floor to utilize their full power.

3 When lifting weights from the floor, keep a natural arch in your back. Pull in your abdominals to support your spine, and never lock your knees.

4 When lifting a weight above your head, never let the weight move behind your head.

5 During sit-ups and crunches, avoid pulling or jerking your neck forward with your hands. Use your hands only to support the weight of your head — lift your head, neck, and shoulders as one unit.

6 When performing abdominal exercises do not anchor your feet. Using sit-up boards with supports for the feet, or having a partner hold your feet, engages the hip flexor muscles and increases the stress on your lower back.

7 Use higher reps in abdominal training to build endurance. Because your abdominals are postural muscles and used in many daily activities, they need to be strong to provide constant support for the spine.

8 Along with exercise to strengthen the abdominal muscles, make sure you also stretch the muscles in the lower back and hamstrings to maintain muscular balance.

9 Give equal time to back extension exercises when doing abdominal training.

10 To better protect your back, do not use excessive weight on exercise machines. One reason weight training machines are popular is that they can isolate limbs but do not require the back muscles to stabilize. Too much reliance on these machines often does more harm than good. Also, the seated posture used on many of these machines can increase pressure on the discs — just the act of sitting increases disc pressure by 40 percent.

Use these simple techniques to avoid needless injuries that may slow you down. You'll not only improve the quality of your workouts, but you'll stay on the cutting edge of fitness, as well.

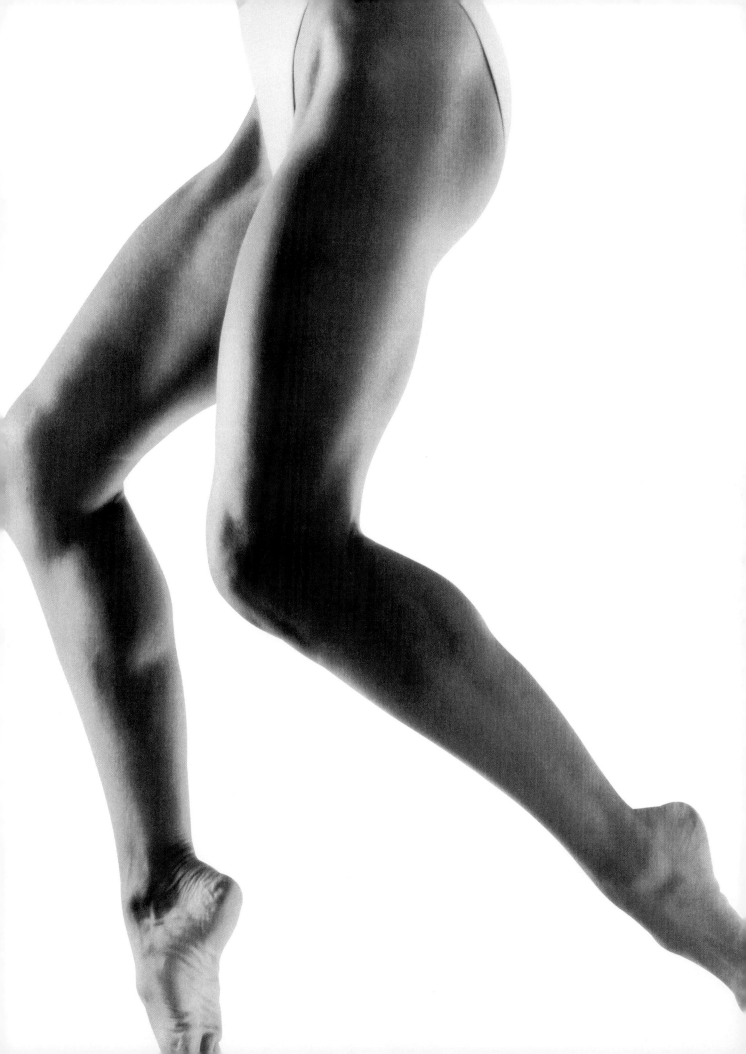

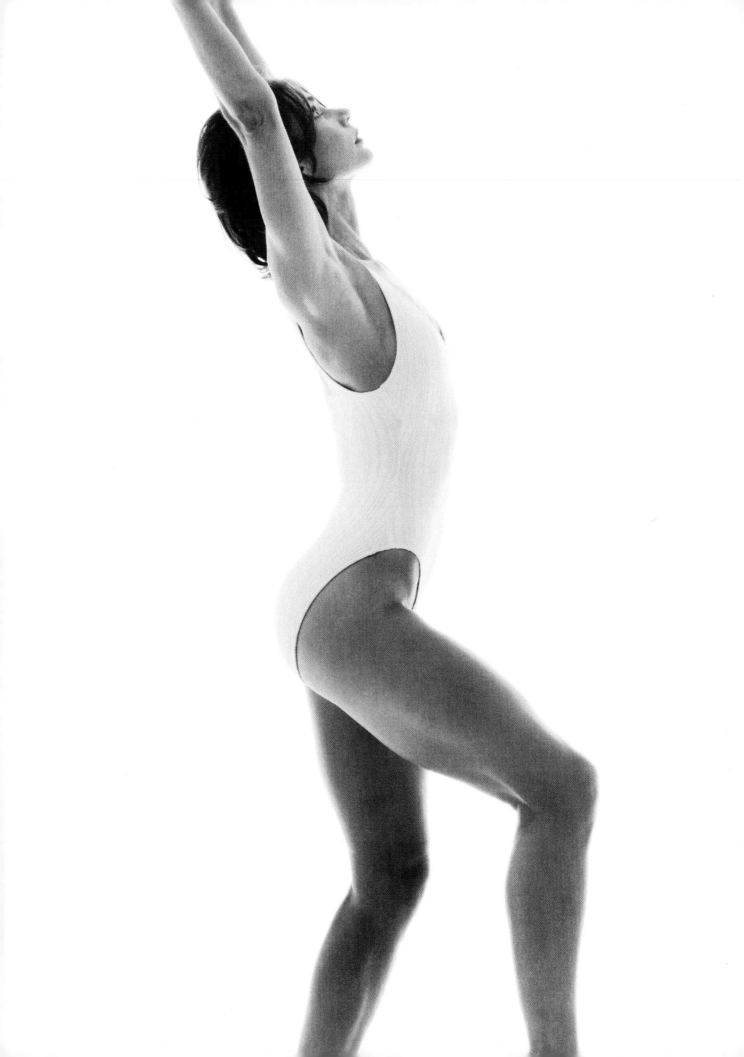

HAVING it all

THE BIGGEST ROADBLOCKS to your success will not be monumental obstacles, but will be the day-to-day interruptions and negative thinking that can sabotage your progress. It may begin with an unrealistic expectation, then become compounded by a hectic day that throws things off schedule. But unless these little stumbling blocks are recognized in advance and addressed with an anticipated response, they accumulate, slow you down, and cause you to give up on even the best laid fitness plans.

Consider Ashley Drake, a successful real estate agent who decided that she'd had enough of the 15 extra pounds she'd gained with the birth of her second child. Her daughter had turned three, and most of her excuses about having to stay home with the baby were gone. With all the good intentions of a goal-oriented achiever, Ashley joined a health club and gave herself six weeks to lose the 15 pounds of "baby fat." The next day Ashley went to the mall and began the task of selecting workout wear. Looking at herself in the mirror, she thought of how she looked five years ago and how she would look in six weeks. She then bought expensive cross-trainer athletic shoes and six exercise outfits. | The next morning she dropped her toddler off at the day-care center and drove eight miles to her new club. After signing in, she was assigned a trainer who set up a weight program for her that was supposed to address her goal. She didn't really like working on the weight machines, nor did she understand the exercises, but she felt too intimidated to say anything. When she left that day, she grabbed an aerobics schedule and planned to make the morning class, thinking she might enjoy this more. | Unfortunately, Ashley's daughter was fussy the next morning and was running a temperature. Ashley decided to skip the morning class and called the office to say that even though she had a heavy work load and that it would be inconvenient, she would work from home. At about 3 P.M. Ashley went to check the fridge for her now very overdue lunch, and later found herself staring into the empty carton of what used to be double-chocolate ice cream. She could hardly believe she'd eaten it all, but chocolate was her downfall. Oh well, she thought, tomorrow's workout would take care of it. | Over the next few days she was frantically trying to catch up with work and pushed gym time to the bottom of the list. Five days later, she crept into the back row of an intermediate/advanced aerobics class and found herself tired and confused by the routine, feeling as if she was a step behind everyone else. She looked in the mirror and felt extremely self-conscious in her colorful workout wear, compared to the skinny girl wearing black who stood next to her. Too discouraged to finish, she left the class 15 minutes early, making up her mind to give the stairclimber a try the next day. The following morning she woke up early and went to the gym, only to find all the stairclimbers occupied. Since she knew she was in for a wait, she went to the juice bar for a breakfast muffin. Even through this was not part of her diet, she thought it would be OK since she was about to work it off. Spotting a free machine, she got on and began her workout. After 10 minutes of stair climbing she became very bored. She noticed a friend of hers walking in and took the opportunity to jump off the stairclimber for a friendly cup of coffee. | The next morning, another friend called and suggested a totally decadent Italian dinner. Italian being Ashley's "other" food nemesis, she felt the offer too tempting to pass up. She stayed on the phone 45 minutes, updating her friend on all the news, including her new exercise program. When she looked at the clock she knew she'd have to run to get to the gym in time. She might not even have time. "Oh what the heck, I'll go tomorrow," she decided, and went back to talking on the phone. | Over the course of the next three weeks, Ashley made it to the gym several times, but felt out of place and disinterested. She weighed two pounds more than when she'd started the program. By week four she had lost all her enthusiasm. By the time her six-week goal came and went, Ashley had abandoned her fitness program with a sense of relief. | Months later when her husband made a well-intentioned comment that she had "put on a few pounds" and suggested she go to the health club, Ashley shrugged and reminded him that she had tried that, but the program didn't work. "I guess it's in my genes—I have exercise-resistant fat," she said. In her mind, the one attempt at exercise had been so negative that she couldn't imagine ever trying it again.

WHAT WENT WRONG

SCHEDULE CHANGES You can't always plan your day around your workouts, so you have to anticipate sick children, work schedule changes, and other interruptions. When your planned schedule gets thrown out of whack, put the brakes on. Instead of abandoning your workout, be prepared to do it at a different time and a different day. This is precisely the kind of day you truly need it. Skipping your workout will only leave you less in control and more stressed. When you remain committed to your workout despite the unexpected schedule changes, you will definitely come out the winner—you'll reenergize yourself and reduce the stress of an out-of-control workday.

If you have to skip a workout it's not the end of your program. Be creative and replace your workout with another activity. Call a friend, or exercise with a family member. If you have only 10 minutes, you can always schedule in a quick calorie-burning activity. Experts have proven that several 10-minute bouts of exercise spread throughout the day can have the accumulated effect of a 20-, 30-, or 40-minute session. Turn your coffee break into a 10-minute brisk walk. Take the stairs two at a time, then turn around and do it again. Polish off the 10 minutes with a brisk walk. Pull out a jump rope at home and do a 10-minute workout. March in place for 10 minutes while dinner is cooking. Everyone can find 10 minutes during their day.

HESITATION It's OK to think about not working out. All of us do. But when this happens, make a conscious effort to think about the rewards from your program. Make a deal with yourself to try just the first five minutes of exercise. After that, if you still don't want to exercise you can quit. More than likely you'll continue. Then reward yourself with a positive thought and acknowledge each workout as a solid step toward your goal. Take pleasure in each small success and realize that a healthy lifestyle is an ongoing process — so enjoy it!

ENTICING OFFERS FROM FRIENDS Let's assume the best — your friends don't *really* intend to sabotage your fitness program, but they do call with enticing plans for dinner or a movie on the spur of the moment, leaving you to decide whether to accept or stick with your workout plan.

Instead of abandoning the program, try to do both! Always keep in mind that abandoning your workout will leave you feeling guilty, especially when you substitute it with a heavily caloric dinner. Ask your friend to meet you an hour later and squeeze in that workout before you indulge. You'll feel great and have fun with your friends too. Or, how about asking your friend to enjoy a workout with you, and then socialize.

DON'T BE TOO HARD ON YOURSELF Once Ashley's program started falling apart, her enthusiasm waned. Within a few days she had a hard time feeling good about herself. Give yourself a little time to find what works for you. Don't get discouraged if you have to try a lot of things before something clicks. Adopting an "all or nothing" attitude early on in the program isn't giving yourself a fair chance.

DON'T COMPARE YOURSELF TO OTHERS The only true measure of your progress is comparing your activity level now to what it was before you began exercising. Don't fall into the trap of comparing yourself to anyone else. Set your own standards. When you see someone in great shape, ask how they do it. Many times you'll find that some of the best bodies out there were out of shape at one time or another.

YOU'RE NOT SEEING RESULTS Make certain that, unlike Ashley, your initial goals are realistic for your schedule and body type. Find a knowledgeable trainer, ask a lot of questions and then make sensible, small, short-term goals.

If you don't see immediate progress, take a step back from your program and really evaluate the situation. Have you truly been giving 100 percent? Have you been consistent? Have you combined your workout with a sensible, healthy, low-fat eating plan? Have you seen mental, emotional, or social benefits that won't show up on the scale or tape measure? Are you feeling better physically and mentally? The likelihood is you have seen progress and are being too hard on yourself. Reevaluate your goals and establish smaller, more incremental goals. For instance, Ashley could have congratulated herself for even trying an intermediate/advanced aerobics class instead of leaving discouraged that she couldn't keep up. Then she could have tried an easier class the next time, feeling even better about herself.

YOU MISS A FEW WEEKS Ok, so you missed a week, two, three, maybe even six weeks of workouts. It's no reason to give up altogether. As a matter of fact, there are advantages to restarting an exercise program. The interim layoff will give you a fresh start and "shock" your muscles into response. You also have the advantage of what exercise enthusiasts call "muscle memory." Once you've worked a muscle or muscle group, it will get back in shape far more quickly than it took to get it in shape the first time. That's a fact. If you abandon your program after only five weeks, you'll be able to get back on track in a matter of two or three. No matter how long you abandon a program, your initial efforts have laid a groundwork from which you can rebuild.

RELATE TO THE PROCESS Remember to enjoy the process of exercising. If the entire time you're exercising you're thinking about when you'll be through, it's hard to stick with a routine. Unlike Ashley, take the time to research exercise. Find a program you like, and learn how the exercise will help you accomplish your goals. Keep yourself informed and you'll feel more confident about your effort. If you find yourself getting bored, approach it like a skill and concentrate on using technique.

OUTSMART YOUR FOOD CRAVINGS Not only did Ashley fail miserably at starting an exercise program, she was ignoring the other half of the equation: good nutrition. Worse, her fallen self-esteem was causing her to indulge her cravings.

When an irresistible urge hits you to eat something that is absolutely off your diet, try these simple craving-busters:

1 Stop and think. Ask yourself if you are really hungry. Is this food really what you want to eat? If the answer is yes to both questions, then just help yourself to a nibble. If the answer is no, then switch gears and identify the specific craving. If it's something sweet, satisfy your chocolate craving with hard candy instead of calorie-rich ice cream. Want something crunchy? How about popcorn instead of potato chips? Chewy? Skip the caramels and try a sports energy bar instead.

2 Break the habit. Instead of giving in to your craving, make a phone call, go shopping, or get up and take a walk outside in the fresh air. Move to another room (not the kitchen) and engage in an activity to take your mind off food. Try putting your favorite quotes on your fridge to keep you mentally motivated and your willpower strong.

3 Ride the wave. Remind yourself that this feeling will pass. Psychologists often compare cravings to the motion of a wave—it begins slowly, builds, and eventually crests and subsides on the beach. Ride out your cravings and they really will go away.

4 Small and slow. It's a good habit to always take small bites and chew them slowly; studies have shown that you will eat less and still be satisfied.

5 Eliminate temptation. If you love Wendy's french fries, make it a point not to drive by the Wendy's on your lunch hour. The same strategy works in your kitchen—if you don't stock the tempting foods, you won't eat them.

ALL OF US TRY TO HAVE IT ALL—financial security, social and personal relationships, and the personal satisfaction that comes with a healthy and attractive body. Most people easily balance two out of three; it's a rare individual who balances all three. But when things in your life don't go as planned, you don't give up—you keep on trying. Exercise deserves the same persistence. Anticipate the possible roadblocks to your success—missed workouts, low-energy days, self-doubt, schedule changes, and the inevitable plateaus in progress we all experience. And when you find yourself slipping, remember that it happens to everyone, get back on track, and stay in the game.

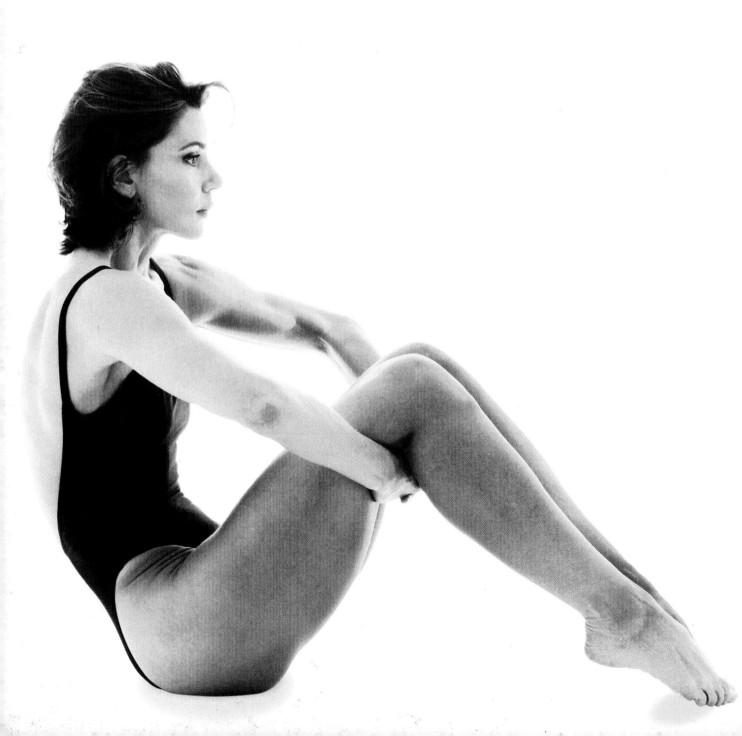

the eating
GAME

WHAT YOU EAT and how much you weigh are intrinsically linked, however, the addition of exercise can work wonders to take the pressure off individuals who simply can't stand to hear the word "diet" one more time. Knowing this makes exercise much more attractive, but you still need to apply certain rules of sensible eating to complement your exercise regime rather than sabotage it.

Moderation is the key. It's what you eat *most* often that counts — slipping up once in a while is not what makes you fat. It's the daily foods you choose that are responsible.

It's also important that you eat what you enjoy. For example, when everyone was claiming pasta was a good choice of low-fat food, I tried eating it in moderate amounts. However, I enjoyed and felt more satisfaction from eating vegetables and lean meats or fish. After having a bowl of pasta, with light sauce, I felt like something was missing. I also got hungry soon after the meal. For me, pasta was not always a good choice for my main meal. Remember that your diet depends on many factors, including lifestyle, genetics, and the rate at which your body requires certain nutrients. It's important to listen to your body, feed it the foods it craves and monitor the amount of fat and calories.

I don't believe in denying yourself foods you crave. Denial tends to lead to binge eating and other unhealthy obsessions. If you simply love chocolate sweets go ahead and enjoy them once in a while — just keep it sensible. If you eat an extra 700 calories of your favorite food try to make up for it with fewer calories and more exercise over the next few days. Also, stop eating before you feel really full.

Think of your body as a fireplace: it needs to be fed substantial fuel to keep it burning throughout the day. If you allow it to burn out, you'll tend to feed it extra to get it going at a steady pace again. This burnout also increases certain cravings, especially quick energy fixes like sugar and caffeine. As evening and bedtime approaches your body needs less fuel; just like a fire that slowly simmers down at night, I eat my biggest meals at breakfast and lunch, and eat only vegetables and fruits after 8 P.M.

SOME FAT IS OK Fat is an essential nutrient. Healthy eating means a *balance* of fat, proteins, and carbohydrates. An overall diet should include some fat but not more than 30 percent. One of the easiest ways to avoid the temptation of high-fat, high-calorie foods is to make them less convenient and accessible. If your kitchen is stocked with healthy foods when that urge to snack strikes, you'll be more likely to nibble on a piece of fruit or rice cake when the ice cream and cookies aren't around. Keeping a good supply of healthy produce in your fridge means you'll always have nutritious alternatives for snacks. Something that works for me is to cut up fresh fruits and attractively arrange them on a plate so I can enjoy them slowly. This feels more like I'm treating myself than it would if I just ate a whole apple. Eating frozen grapes or marinated grilled vegetables is another way I glamorize my snacks.

POWER PRODUCE Here are some simple tips to get more power when shopping in your produce aisle:

• Broccoli is a powerhouse of vitamins and minerals. By many accounts, it is the most nutritious of all vegetables.

• Green peppers are richer in vitamin C than oranges—add them to salads, soups and casseroles.

• Spinach and bok choy top the list of nutritious green leafy vegetables—steam for just two minutes to retain their generous store of nutrients.

• Tomatoes are not only high in potassium and vitamins A and C, they also contain beneficial phytochemicals that may prevent heart disease and cancers.

• Cantaloupes are packed with vitamins, yet are very low in calories. A great breakfast treat.

• Leafy green and yellow or orange vegetables add beta-carotene and vitamin C to your diet.

• Prewashed, packaged salad and stir-fry ingredients save you time preparing fresh vegetables.

• When making salads, skip the croutons, avocados, cheese, and olives.

• Eat fruit for desserts and snacks.

CUT THE FAT: KEEP THE DAIRY Dairy products are an important source of calcium, protein, and riboflavin. However, they are also a source of fat and cholesterol. Try using skim milk whenever possible; it can definitely be included in a smoothie, in oatmeal, and used in recipes requiring whole milk.

Love condiments, cheese, and dips? You don't have to give them up; just be a little nontraditional. Buttermilk is very low in fat and can be used instead of many of the high-fat creams called for in recipes. Also, check out the dairy counter for fat-free and reduced-fat sour cream and cream cheese.

RED MEATS, POULTRY, AND FISH Meats are an excellent source of muscle-building protein. You don't have to completely eliminate red meat—while it can be high in fat it is also high in protein, iron, and zinc. Make certain the cuts you choose are free from marbling or visible fat. Purchase meats marked "lean," "extra lean," or "select" rather than "choice" or "prime" cuts.

Cooking preferable cuts of meat in liquid, such as red wine, will make them more tender. Skinless poultry, especially the white meat of the breast, is very low in fat while high in protein. If you buy cooked poultry with the skin on, make sure you remove it before eating.

While many fish are high in oils and fat, they are also high in HDL, the "good" cholesterol, making them an excellent choice in a healthy diet. Eat water-packed tuna, salmon, and sardines for a healthy heart and a great protein source.

CARBOHYDRATES: WHICH ARE BEST?

Everyone needs a generous supply of carbohydrates in their diet to provide fuel for activities. As always, try to eat foods as close to their natural state as possible: unrefined, raw, and lightly cooked foods are nearly always more nutritious than processed foods. For your daily carbs, take your pick from potatoes, rice, couscous, bulgur, and whole wheat products and eat them early in the day. Serve them with lean meat, fish, or vegetables in a stir-fry as your main dish. My favorite way to eat carbs during the day is to prepare a potato this way: I wash a medium-sized russet potato, and put it in a fold-top or resealable plastic food-storage bag, and cook it in a microwave oven on high for 12 minutes. Then I leave it in the bag so the steam heat continues to cook the potato slowly. I throw it in my purse when I leave for work, and by lunchtime, I have a perfectly cooked, moist baked potato that's still warm. Doing this first thing in the morning while I'm getting dressed is a great time-saver and gives me something nutritious to eat on those hectic days.

Don't forget the beans — chick-peas, lentils, kidney, and other dried beans are excellent sources of protein and carbohydrates and rich in B vitamins. Load them on salads or mix with other vegetables.

CAN YOU GET FAT ON NO-FAT?

With so much talk about low-fat diets, it seems that some people misinterpreted nutritionists who were saying eat a "sensible, low-fat diet," and instead heard "eat all you want, as long as it's low-fat or nonfat." Thus, people found themselves gaining weight on pasta and the endless variety of nonfat foods that fill our grocery store shelves. Remember that a calorie is still a calorie, whether it's from fat or carbohydrates. If you eat more calories than you burn, those extra calories are stored as fat. It's as simple as that.

FROZEN FOODS, QUICK SOUPS, AND SNACKS

In today's fast-paced world, frozen foods and dehydrated soups are a big part of many people's diets. Select dishes that do not have sauces. Try to keep sodium at less than 500 mg. per meal. Pass up the breaded meats and fish. In the ice cream freezer, look for sorbet or nonfat frozen yogurt.

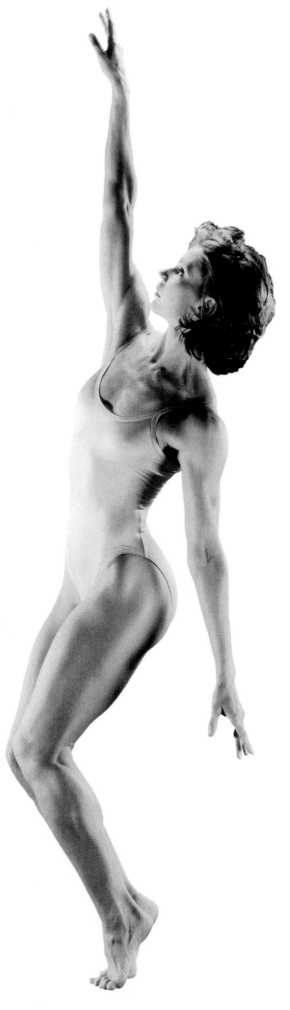

There's nothing wrong with instant soup, but read labels and beware of the salt, msg, oil, and cream bases they may contain. Even chicken soup can be loaded with salt and fat.

As far as low-fat snacks go, everyone has their favorite. Mine is red licorice vines. You might also try pretzels, rice cakes, air-popped pop-corn, angel food cake, or ginger snaps. And if you want to be really good, cut up some fresh celery, bell peppers, and carrots for snacks. Whatever route you choose, make certain you eat snacks in moderation.

THE LOW-FAT GOURMET   Contrary to some beliefs, you can cut the fat and still retain the flavor. Check the condiment aisle for some of the wonderful new twists on regular mustard, then use them instead of mayonnaise or butter to spice up sandwiches.

Bake, broil, or poach, but never fry. Sauté foods in white or red wine or in chicken broth. If you want to, use a small amount of olive oil, not butter or margarine. I love to use cooking spray for just the perfect amount.

SEVEN SENSIBLE MENUS Wondering how to eat sensibly?
Here's a week-long diet to get you started. You can drink all the
water you like. Between meals you can snack on fresh fruit, raw
vegetables, and rice cakes.

MONDAY

BREAKFAST
- Oatmeal topped with
  sliced fresh fruit
- 1 low-fat bran muffin
- Coffee or tea

LUNCH
- Mixed green salad with
  1T salad dressing topped
  with water-packed tuna
  (3¼ oz.)
- 3 whole grain crackers
- Fat-free beverage
- ½ cup Italian ice or sorbet

DINNER
- Grilled skinless chicken breast
- 1 cup seasoned steamed
  green beans
- Steamed red potatoes
  sprinkled with a little
  cayenne pepper and
  Mrs. Dash
- ½ cup frozen nonfat yogurt
- Fat-free beverage

TUESDAY

BREAKFAST
- Fruit juice
- 2 whole wheat pancakes
  with 2T maple syrup
- ½ cup berries on top
- Nonfat flavored yogurt
- Coffee or tea

LUNCH
- Pita bread stuffed with 3 oz.
  chicken, lettuce, tomato, and
  chopped celery
- 1 cup low-fat pasta salad
- Fat-free beverage
- ½ cup fruit and gelatin

DINNER
- Grilled whitefish with lemon
- Caesar salad with
  1T salad dressing
- Grilled zucchini halves
- 3 ginger snaps

WEDNESDAY

BREAKFAST
- Fruit juice
- Bran flakes with nonfat milk
  and sliced banana
- 1 toasted english muffin
- Coffee or tea

LUNCH
- 2 slices of roasted
  turkey breast
- 1 large baked potato stuffed
  with steamed vegetables and
  1T creamy dressing
- Small bunch of grapes
- 1 nonfat beverage

DINNER
- Steamed potstickers
- Stir-fried beef or chicken
  with broccoli and onion,
  mushrooms, and snowpeas
- Steamed rice
- Orange slices with
  fortune cookie

THURSDAY

BREAKFAST
- Fruit juice
- 2-3 scrambled egg whites with spinach and mushrooms
- 1-2 toasted bran cakes with 2T jam
- Coffee or tea

LUNCH
- Lean roast beef sandwich: 2 oz. beef on sourdough roll with lettuce, tomato, and mustard
- ½ cup carrot/raisin salad
- 2 fig-filled cookies
- Fat-free beverage

DINNER
- Grilled lemon chicken breast
- Dinner salad with 1T salad dressing
- Steamed asparagus
- Slice of angel food cake topped with raspberries or strawberries
- Fat-free beverage

FRIDAY

BREAKFAST
- Fruit juice
- Wedge of honeydew
- 7 grain or oatbran muffin
- Coffee or tea

LUNCH
- Vegetable soup
- Voight Chicken Salad*
- Fresh peach, orange, or apple
- Fat free beverage

DINNER
- 3 oz. broiled cod or halibut
- Steamed kale with lightly sautéed, chopped onions and garlic
- ½ cup basmati rice
- ½ cup sorbet with diced fresh fruit
- Fat-free beverage

SATURDAY

BREAKFAST
- Fruit juice
- Unsweetened ready-to-eat cereal with sliced strawberries and ½ cup nonfat milk
- ½ papaya with a squeeze of lime
- 1 slice toast with jam
- Coffee or tea

LUNCH
- Turkey breast sandwich on rye bread with mustard, tomato, and lettuce
- Tossed green salad with 1T dressing
- Sliced yellow and red bell pepper rings
- Watermelon wedge

DINNER
- Grilled shrimp and scallop kabobs with nonfat Italian salad dressing marinade
- ½ cup couscous
- Grilled vegetables
- 1 scoop sorbet served in ½ cantaloupe
- Fat-free beverage

SUNDAY

BREAKFAST
- Fruit juice
- 2 frozen whole-grain low-fat waffles topped with ½ cup blueberries and 1T maple syrup
- 1 cup mixed fresh fruit salad
- Coffee or tea

LUNCH
- Voight Chicken Tacos*
- Sliced cucumber salad with rice vinegar

DINNER
- Marinated Flank Steak*
- Corn on the cob
- Arugula salad with sliced tomatoes and 1T salad dressing
- Baked cinnamon apple

*see recipes on pages 126–127

VOIGHT'S RECIPES

VOIGHT CHICKEN SALAD

3T red vinegar

1T dark sesame oil

½ t. crushed red pepper

1 (2¼ pounds) whole roasted chicken, skinned

½ cup fresh cilantro leaves

1 clove crushed garlic

2T sesame seeds, toasted

1 (10-ounce) bag prepackaged
European salad greens (about 6 cups)

Combine first 3 ingredients in a large bowl; stir well, and set aside. Remove chicken from the bones and shred with 2 forks to measure about 4 cups of meat. Add chicken, cilantro, garlic, sesame seeds, and greens to the dressing bowl, and toss gently to coat. Serve immediately.

Serves 4: 282 calories; 35 grams protein; 14 grams fat; 2.5 grams carbohydrate

MARINATED FLANK STEAK

¼ cup lemon juice

2 t. dried rosemary leaves, crushed

2 garlic cloves, crushed

3 t. low sodium soy sauce

1 flank steak (1 to 1¼ pounds)

2 cups cooked fettuccine noodles

2 cups steamed green beans with
red bell peppers and onions

In a self-sealing plastic bag, combine lemon juice, water, rosemary, garlic, and bouillon; mix well. Add steak; seal bag. Marinate 6 hours or overnight, turning occasionally.

Use a barbecue or preheat broiler. Remove meat from marinade; transfer marinade to small pan and put on medium-high heat until it comes to a boil; reduce heat and simmer 2 minutes. Place steak on grill or broiler pan. Grill or broil 15 minutes, basting frequently with marinade.

To serve, slice steak thinly and accompany with fettuccine and green beans.

Serves 5: 475 calories; 30 grams protein; 18 grams fat; 50 grams carbohydrates

VOIGHT CHICKEN TACOS

4 (4-ounce) skinned, boned chicken breast halves

2 t. lemon juice

¼ t. each salt and pepper

4 (8 in.) corn tortillas

Vegetable cooking spray

1 t. vegetable oil

2 green onions, cut into ¼-inch slices

½ cup low-fat sour cream mixed with

¼ cup plain nonfat yogurt

1 cup fresh or low-sodium salsa

3 cups shredded lettuce

Fresh cilantro sprigs

Place the chicken in a shallow dish. Combine the lemon juice, salt, and pepper in a small bowl and pour it over the chicken. Cover and chill 30 minutes. Wrap the tortillas in foil and bake at 325 degrees for 10–15 minutes or until heated.

Coat a large nonstick skillet with cooking spray and heat over medium-high heat until hot. Add the chicken and cook 6 minutes on each side until chicken is done. Remove and drain; pat dry with paper towels. Cut the chicken into ½-inch cubes; set aside.

Heat the oil in a skillet over medium-high heat. Add the green onions and cook 1 minute or until tender. Return the chicken to the skillet; cook until thoroughly heated. Remove from the heat and stir in ¼ cup each sour cream and yogurt.

Spoon the chicken mixture onto the tortillas; top with the salsa. Roll up the tortillas. Serve each one on ¾ cup shredded lettuce and top with 1 tablespoon of sour cream. Garnish with fresh cilantro sprigs.

Serves 4: 313 calories; 32 grams protein; 9 grams fat; 19 grams carbohydrates

20 most-asked questions

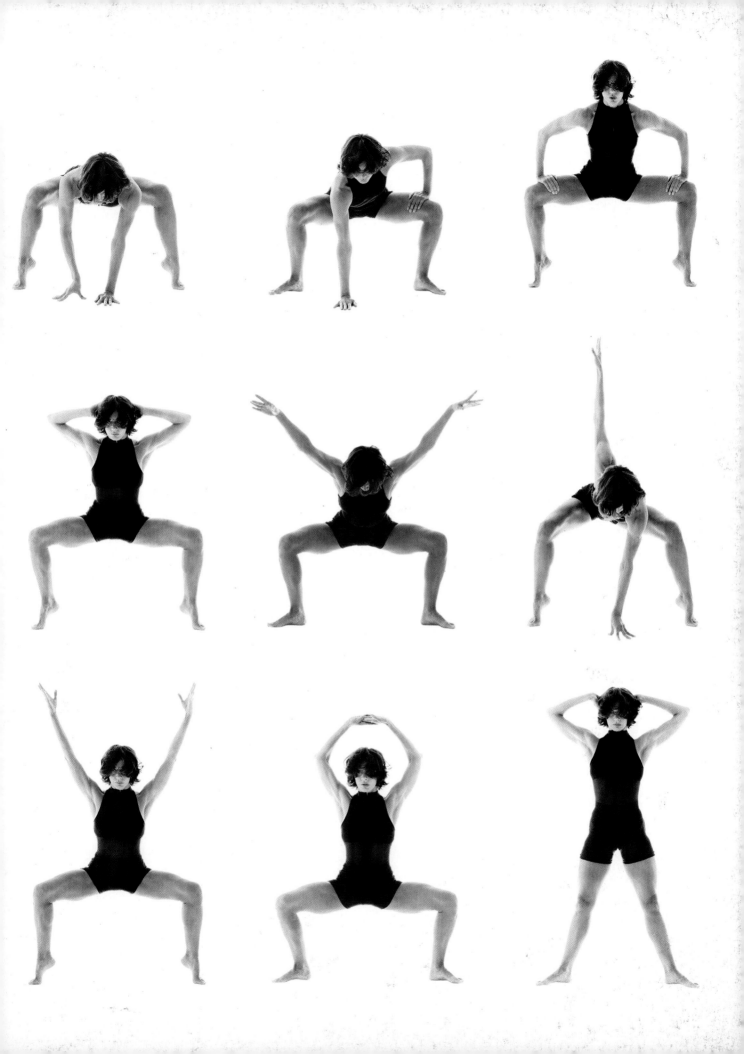

1 I'VE NEVER EXERCISED BEFORE BUT I WANT TO START EXERCISING. HOW DO I BEGIN?

To start any fitness program, begin with walking. Start with five or ten minutes, then increase by one- or two-minute increments building up to a 20- or 30-minute walk on a consistent basis.

Begin the precision training exercises, use limited range of motion and sufficient rest between the exercises. Do only what feels comfortable.

If you feel fatigued, slow down, take a break, then resume at your own pace. You will burn more calories by taking it slow, for a longer duration, than you will by pushing yourself hard for a short amount of time.

2 HOW MUCH AND HOW OFTEN SHOULD I EXERCISE?

Try to fit in some aerobic activity every day. Along with aerobics, you can do my precision workout for 20 to 30 minutes up to five times per week. Most people, find that three to four days a week is sufficient.

If you are short of time, exercise experts estimate the minimum time you should spend exercising is 20 to 30 minutes, three times a week, to impart a noticeable training benefit. New research proves that even ten-minute bouts of exercise, scattered throughout your day, can improve your fitness level.

3 WHAT EQUIPMENT DO I NEED?

As you progress in a routine you may require more gear, but to begin you need only:

- Hand weights; I prefer between two to five pounds
- Ankle weights; I prefer two and a half to five pounds
- A 12-pound Voight bar, padded (optional)
- A 3-pound Voight Ball (optional)

4 HOW DO I CHOOSE THE RIGHT SHOE?

If you're doing aerobic exercise, your shoe may be the most important piece of gear you purchase. It should:

- Be snug, not tight. Remember, your feet will expand with exercise as they get warm.
- Feel comfortable and be free of seams or rough surfaces that can irritate your feet.
- Have flexible soles, particularly in the front or ball of your foot.
- Provide good arch support.
- Fit well: You should be able to wiggle your toes, and you should have a small space between the tip of your longest toe and the inside of the shoe.

Here are some tips to make your shoes last longer:

- When the shoe stretches, wear thicker socks or two pairs to make the fit snug again.

- If your shoes become wet from perspiration, take them off right after the workout and let them air out.
- Purchase a pair of shoes just for exercise — don't walk around in them for daily activities; this will unnecessarily wear out their support and padding.

Here are some tips when you try on the shoes:
- Wear the same kind of socks you'll be wearing when you exercise.
- Try on shoes in the middle of the day.
- Try on both shoes, and walk around in them.

5 WHAT IS THE DIFFERENCE BETWEEN WORKING HARD AND OVER-DOING IT?

There are very distinct feelings associated with each. Basically, when you're working hard it's OK to feel:
- A slightly elevated heart rate, which goes back to normal shortly after exercise.
- An increase in breathing, but not so much that you cannot converse in a regular manner of speech.
- A slight stretching or squeezing sensation in the working muscles.
- Mild perspiration.
- Some muscle soreness the day after, but not persisting more than 72 hours.
- Fatigue, but not exhaustion.

The following are symptoms associated with overdoing it, which should signal you to stop exercising, rest, and consider contacting your physician:
- Shortness of breath, difficulty in speech.
- Irregular heartbeat or pulse.
- Pain or discomfort in the chest, neck, or arms.
- Nausea, dizziness, cold sweats.
- Joint pain or chronic muscle ache.

6 I'M COMMITTED BUT NEW TO THIS. DO YOU HAVE POINTERS ON HOW TO BEGIN AN IN-HOME ROUTINE?

Set realistic short-term goals. Use your goal-oriented mind-set to set a small goal for the end of the week.

Next, decide on a specific time to work out and stick with it! Plan a schedule to include your workout rather than letting your schedule exclude your workout plans.

Get everything you need in one place. Open this book to the first workout and place it on your living room floor. If you're doing an aerobics tape, put the tape in the VCR, cued up and ready to go.

Keep an exercise bag filled with everything you'll need: workout wear, shoes and socks, hand weights and a towel. Store other accessories close by.

Place a mirror in your workout area to check your position. Match body positions as closely as you can with what you see in the book or on the screen.

Have water handy. Fill a plastic bottle with water or your favorite recovery drink and have it close at hand.

When you are ready to exercise, turn on the answering machine so that you don't have to worry about interruptions. Tie your hair back, wash your face to feel more energized, and simply begin.

7 WHAT IS THE PURPOSE OF A WARM-UP AND A COOL-DOWN?

The exercises prescribed in this book are in a particular order to warm up your muscles, work your muscles, and then cool them down. The warm-up provides a smooth transition from the resting state to the full exertion required at the peak of the movement. At the end of the exercise session, the stretching movements are designed to gradually diminish tension and allow your body to go back to its restive state. This will reduce the chance that you will experience muscle soreness following the workout.

8 WHAT IS THE DIFFERENCE BETWEEN MUSCULAR STRENGTH AND MUSCULAR ENDURANCE?

Muscular strength is the maximum force a muscle can generate. That means a grit-your-teeth kind of exertion that bodybuilders and weightlifters train with in order to stimulate maximum muscular growth and strength.

Muscular endurance, on the other hand, is the ability of the muscle to make repeated contractions against a less-than-maximal load. This is what is required in cycling, running, skating, and aerobic dance.

In general, it is believed that both types of benefit should be elicited from exercise. Some people may desire higher levels than others because of certain pursuits, making it difficult to assign a particular ratio to a given individual. The program prescribed in this book imparts a healthy balance of strength and endurance conditioning for the average individual.

9 WHY HAVE I GAINED WEIGHT SINCE I BEGAN WORKING OUT EIGHT WEEKS AGO?

Many people experience an initial weight gain when they begin to exercise because they are adding muscle. Muscle is more dense than other tissue and weighs more. Therefore, you can decrease fat and increase muscle, and even though you are physically smaller than you were before you began exercising, you may actually weigh more on the scale.

10 IS IT POSSIBLE TO SPOT REDUCE?

In theory there is no such thing as spot reduction. However, just as your body gains and stores fat disproportionately, you may lose more fat from one area than another. Unfortunately, the newest fat gained is usually the first to go, and most people desire to rid themselves of "old" fat, particularly the fat on the thighs, buttocks, and abdomen. The good news is that with a consistent program, even the most stubborn lower body fat will begin to disappear. Putting extra effort into training the lower body will improve muscle tone there and will also contribute to a greater number of calories burned due to the fact that you will be working large muscle groups.

11 HOW DO I EAT HEALTHY WHEN EATING OUT?

Always order salad dressing on the side and use no more than one or two tablespoons. Order light or no-fat dressings. When this isn't possible, mix the regular dressing with vinegar or lemon juice. Try mixing vinegar with a sugar substitute—it makes a sweet dressing with almost no calories or fat. Also:

- Never order fried foods.
- Order lean cuts of meat—white poultry without the skin and fish are excellent. Avoid cream-based sauces and all gravies.
- Avoid appetizers and buffet foods—both are usually high in fat.

- At Asian restaurants, order lots of vegetables and steamed rice to fill you up.
- Request that the chef use only minimal oil and no butter in preparation.
- If you want dessert, order fruit, low-fat yogurt, sorbet, angel food cake, or another healthy dessert.

12 I CAN HANDLE MOST THINGS ABOUT LOW-FAT EATING, BUT I SIMPLY CAN'T STOMACH A BAKED POTATO WITH NOTHING ON IT! WHAT DO I DO?

Try sour cream instead of butter or margarine. Tablespoon for tablespoon, sour cream has 75 percent less fat. Ask for it on the side, and use no more than one tablespoon. Salsa can also spice up your potato without adding any unnecessary fat.

13 I'M NO MATH WHIZ SO JUST GIVE IT TO ME STRAIGHT: HOW MANY GRAMS OF FAT CAN I HAVE A DAY?

Don't eat more than 3 grams of fat for every 100 calories you consume. That means if you eat an average of 2,000 calories a day, don't eat more than 60 grams of fat a day.

14 I'M PREGNANT. WHAT SPECIAL PRECAUTIONS DO I NEED TO TAKE?

Women are encouraged to continue an already

established exercise program when they are pregnant, but each individual should consult her physician to assess her particular needs. If you have not exercised prior to becoming pregnant, you should not begin an exercise program until consulting your physician.

According to the American College of Obstetricians and Gynecologists, you should:

- Exercise three days per week, with warm-up and cool-down.
- Avoid exercising in hot or humid weather.
- Avoid any activity that causes your heart rate to go above 140 beats per minute.
- Avoid exercises that require you to lie on your back after the fourth month.
- Avoid extreme strength exercises and movements that require deep flexion or extension.

15 SOME DAYS I HAVE TROUBLE FOCUSING ON MY EXERCISE. WHAT DO I DO?

Before you start, try washing your face and rinsing with cool water. This helps energize you and creates a fresh state of mind. When you begin exercising, listen to your body. Remember that breath control can be a tremendous help in maximizing your progress and focusing energy. Make a point of exhaling on the effort. Make a clear and conscious effort to focus and direct your energies on the movement, and don't daydream!

16 WHAT IS TARGET HEART RATE?

The best way to measure the intensity of exercise is to check your heart rate during the activity. As a result of scientific study you can now estimate the appropriate level of intensity, called your Target Heart Rate or THR. The THR is actually a zone providing you a range of heart rates that are high enough to provide a training effect, but low enough to allow you to exercise safely for 20 to 60 minutes.

17 HOW DO I DETERMINE MY THR?

First, you need to monitor your heart rate. This is done by counting the pulse rate at your neck or wrist for ten seconds (if using the wrist, use your first two fingers, not your thumb, to count). Always take your pulse immediately following exercise, within five seconds, because your heart rate falls quickly. The following chart, adapted from Howley and Franks (1986) shows your THR based on this 10-second count:

AGE	BEGINNING beats/10 sec	INTERMEDIATE beats/10 sec	ADVANCED beats/10 sec
-19	20-24	23-25	25-29
20-24	20-24	23-25	24-29
25-29	18-22	22-25	24-29
30-34	18-22	22-25	24-29
35-39	18-21	21-23	22-26
40-44	16-21	20-23	21-25
45-49	16-20	20-22	21-25
50-54	15-19	19-22	20-23
55-59	15-19	19-21	18-23
60+	15-18	18-21	16-22

18 I'D LIKE TO DO A WALK-RUN PROGRAM. ANY SUGGESTIONS?

Here are some safe guidelines to begin:

- Always begin with walking for your warm-up.
- Begin with a 10-step run, 10-step walk. Increase your run by ten steps, until you are running for more than a minute. Then increase your running time by minutes. Alternate your running time with a 10-step walk.
- Progress slowly, never moving to the next level unless you are comfortable.
- Keep your THR at the low end of the zone.
- Begin your program with one day on, one day off.
- Stay aware of your body and the development of any new aches and pains.

19 I'D LIKE TO USE SWIMMING AS MY AEROBIC ACTIVITY. ANY ADVICE?

Swimming is an excellent form of exercise. Here are some pointers if you are just getting back into swimming:

- If available, chest-deep water is ideal.
- Begin by walking or jogging the width of the pool several times. Check that you are within your THR, if not, continue walking and jogging until your conditioning level is up.

- Begin by swimming one length, and walking back, checking that you are within your THR. Increase the duration of continuous swimming until you can accomplish 20 to 30 minutes without a rest. By swimming every other day you will be enjoying one of the finest and safest forms of aerobic activity.

20 I'D LIKE TO USE CYCLING AS MY AEROBIC ACTIVITY. ANY GUIDELINES?

Cycling—whether outdoors or indoors on a stationary bike—is an invigorating aerobic activity that concentrates on the lower body and burns maximum calories. When you start:

- If you are not conditioned for cycling, begin by riding one or two miles, three times per week.
- Gradually increase the distance and time. Your first workouts may be just ten minutes in duration, but this will change quickly. In five-minute increments, increase your duration until you can easily peddle for 30 to 60 minutes and stay within your THR.

SAVE $5.00
BY MAIL WHEN YOU BUY

THE #1 FITNESS VIDEO OF THE YEAR ...AND THE ULTIMATE FITNESS GUIDE!

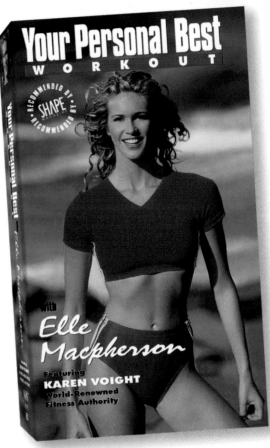

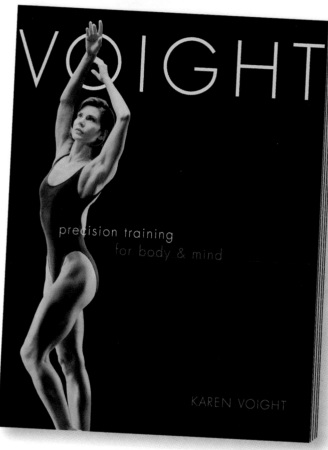

- The #1 video on Billboard magazine's 1995 fitness video charts!
- Recommended by Shape magazine!
- Perfectly timed for pre-swimsuit season!
- Features a uniquely entertaining and effective workout developed by fitness expert Karen Voight!

- Written by IDEA Fitness Instructor Of The Year Karen Voight!
- It's the ultimate guide to total fitness of body, mind and spirit!
- Designed to enhance, inspire and strengthen women at <u>any</u> fitness level!
- Addresses <u>all</u> aspects of fitness, including stretching, nutrition and motivation!

"Karen Voight is a powerhouse in the fitness industry! She has designed a solid total-body workout that's believable, easy to follow, and has great athletic appeal!"

—SHAPE MAGAZINE

Consult with your doctor before beginning this or any exercise routine.

Offer good on YOUR PERSONAL BEST WORKOUT WITH ELLE MACPHERSON video only. Offer not good on Karen Voight fitness videos distributed by ABC Home Video.

Buena Vista Home Video   © Buena Vista Home Video, Inc.   [CC]

Here's How The Powerful Combination of Karen And Elle Can Help You Get Your $5 Refund!

BUY: *Your Personal Best Workout With Elle Macpherson* video and *Voight Total Precision For Body And Mind* book.

SEND:
1) This original, hand-printed certificate (no photocopies).
2) Proof-of-purchase tab from *Your Personal Best Workout With Elle Macpherson* AND your cash register receipt (printed with store name and the price you paid for your video) dated between April 15, 1996, and April 15, 1998 (photocopy of receipt is acceptable) for your video purchase.
3) The cash register receipt printed with store name and the price you paid for your *Voight Total Precision For Body And Mind* book circled. Receipt must be dated between April 15, 1996, and April 15, 1998.

RECEIVE: A refund check for $5.00.

LIMIT: FIVE $5.00 REFUNDS PER NAME OR ADDRESS.

MAIL TO: *Your Personal Best Workout With Elle Macpherson* $5.00 Refund, P.O. Box 2641, Maple Plain, MN 55592-2641

Name: _____ Phone #: (_____) _____

Address: _____ Apt. #: _____

City: _____ State/Province: _____ Zip/Postal Code: _____

Offer valid, and purchases must be made, between April 15, 1996, and April 15, 1998. Store receipts must emanate from same state/province as consumer address. Group entries void. Refunds will not be mailed to P.O. Boxes. Check with your local post office for a street address. Refund rights may not be assigned or transferred. Requests not in compliance with the terms of this offer will not be acknowledged or returned. Multiple submissions are subject to verification. Use of multiple addresses or P.O. Boxes to obtain additional refunds is fraud and may result in prosecution. This form is required and must accompany your request. This form and proof-of-purchase tabs may not be reproduced in any manner. Any requests for offer forms mailed to this P.O. Box number or Buena Vista Home Video will not be acknowledged. Offer good in U.S.A. and Canada. Void where prohibited, restricted, or taxed by law. Please allow 8-12 weeks for delivery. Inquiries regarding this offer received later than 6 months after the expiration date will not be acknowledged. PRINTED IN U.S.A.

MIRAMAX HOME ENTERTAINMENT

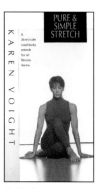
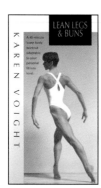
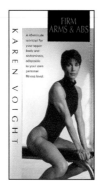
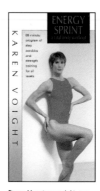
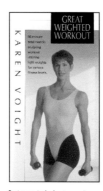
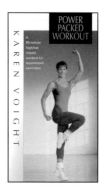
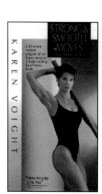

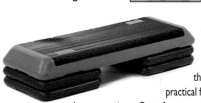
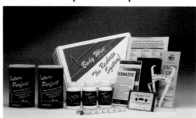